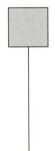

CANCER IN
YOUNG ADULTS

FACING DEATH

Series editor: David Clark, Professor of Medical Sociology,
University of Sheffield

The subject of death in late modern culture has become a rich field of theoretical, clinical and policy interest. Widely regarded as a taboo until recent times, death now engages a growing interest among social scientists, practitioners and those responsible for the organization and delivery of human services. Indeed, how we die has become a powerful commentary on how we live and the specialized care of dying people holds an important place within modern health and social care.

This series captures such developments. Among the contributors are leading experts in death studies, from sociology, anthropology, social psychology, ethics, nursing, medicine and pastoral care. A particular feature of the series is its attention to the developing field of palliative care, viewed from the perspectives of practitioners, planners and policy analysts; here several authors adopt a multi disciplinary approach, drawing on recent research, policy and organizational commentary, and reviews of evidence-based practice. Written in a clear, accessible style, the entire series will be essential reading for students of death, dying and bereavement and for anyone with an involvement in palliative care research, service delivery or policy-making.

Current and forthcoming titles:

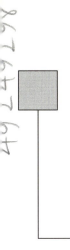

CANCER IN
YOUNG ADULTS
Through parents' eyes

ANNE GRINYER

OPEN UNIVERSITY PRESS
Buckingham · Philadelphia

Open University Press
Celtic Court
22 Ballmoor
Buckingham
MK18 1XW

email: enquiries@openup.co.uk
world wide web: www.openup.co.uk

and
325 Chestnut Street
Philadelphia, PA 19106, USA

First Published 2002

A catalogue record of this book is available from the British Library

ISBN 0 335 21230 1 (pb)   0 335 21231 X (hb)

Library of Congress Cataloging-in-Publication Data
Grinyer, Anne, 1950–
    Cancer in young adults: through parents' eyes / Anne Grinyer.
        p. cm. – (Facing death)
    Includes bibliographical references and index.
    ISBN 0-335-21230-1 (pb) – ISBN 0-335-21230-1 (hb)
    1. Tumors in adolescence. I. Title. II. Series.
RC281.C4 G77 2002
616.99′4′00835–dc21
                                                            2002022772

Typeset by Graphicraft Limited, Hong Kong
Printed in Great Britain by St Edmundsbury Press, Bury St Edmunds, Suffolk

This book is dedicated to the memory of George, and to all of the young people whose stories are told.

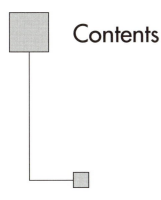

Contents

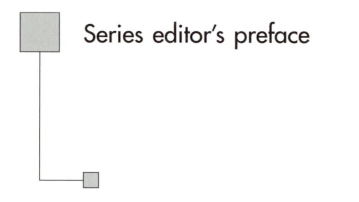

Series editor's preface

It was at Lancaster University in December of the year 2000 that I first discussed the idea for this book with Anne Grinyer and Carol Thomas. I was immediately moved by what I heard about their work and gave every encouragement I could to the project. Now that the book is complete I am more than ever convinced of its importance.

In the late modern world the experience of adolescence and young adulthood has become characterized by risk and reflexivity. For many it is an interlude of shifting liminality between a sense of dependency upon the family and household of early life and the prospect of a new found independence. It is a period portrayed as exciting, uncertain and potentially conflictual. This book describes what happens when another element is introduced into this already complex situation. It takes us into the world of young adults who face a life-threatening illness, as seen through the eyes of their parents.

Anne Grinyer has taken this immensely difficult subject matter and forged it into a compassionate and searching book. She offers us the accounts of 28 young people, from the perspectives of their parents, as they first encounter and then move through the narrative of serious illness, in some cases leading to death itself. We are taken through the trajectories of treatment, the encounters with the health care system, the journey of finding meaning. No one will remain unaffected by these accounts, which are set out in such detail by the parents who took part in the study. They provide us with a remarkable window on suffering and are an extraordinary testimony to the human capacity for care, for resilience and hope.

The book deals with challenging topics. There are accounts of sexuality and fertility in the context of terminal illness. There are issues about money. There are decriptions of the reactions of siblings and the management of conflict. Hugely important too, are the analyses of medical involvement and decision-making in the treatment process. We gain access to changing family dynamics, to the search for 'normality' and to the effects on marital relationships. In every case, however, Anne Grinyer has added to these accounts with some wider commentary on the implications for health and social care practitioners. Accordingly, the narratives, whilst redolent with their own moral authority, are also contextualized in the formal care system and can be seen as evidence to support changes in policy and practice.

Cancer in Young Adults combines an ethical integrity with practical relevance. It takes an unusual social science method in which respondents are invited to furnish written accounts of their experience, and applies it to an emotionally challenging subject matter. This combination of methodological innovation and sensitivity is found in other books in the Facing Death series which have used a broadly ethnographic orientation. Examples include an analysis of the management of death in the intensive care unit (Seymour 2001); a study of illness 'calendars' in cancer (Costain Schou and Hewison 1998), and an ethnography of the maintenance of hope among patients in a lung cancer clinic (The 2002). The subject matter explored here is also close to that considered by Riches and Dawson (2000) in their book about bereaved parents and siblings.

Anne Grinyer has written a worthy companion to these volumes. She has also paid a profound tribute to the parents, their sons and daughters, whose experiences are her subject matter. In so many ways too, this is the finest of tributes to the young man who, by his remarkable courage and intellect, inspired not only the idea for this piece of research, but also the hearts and minds of so many others who knew him, or who, like I did, came to know him only after his untimely death.

David Clark

References

Costain Schou, K. and Hewison, J. (1998) *Experiencing Cancer: Quality of Life in Treatment*. Buckingham: Open University Press.

Riches, G. and Dawson, P. (2000) *An Intimate Loneliness: Supporting Bereaved Parents and Siblings*. Buckingham: Open University Press.

Seymour, J. (2001) *Critical Moments: Death and Dying in Intensive Care*. Buckingham: Open University Press.

The, A-M. (2002) *Palliative Care and Communication: Experiences in the Clinic*. Buckingham: Open University Press.

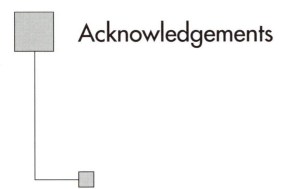

Acknowledgements

There are many people and organizations whose support and advice were valued throughout the project. Thanks go to: The George Easton Memorial Trust for their financial support, and all those who raised money for the Trust thus enabling the research to take place. Myrna Whiteson of The Teenage Cancer Trust and Sue Morgan, Macmillan Nurse, who both confirmed the need for the research and gave encouragement in the early stages. David Clark for his belief in the book and his valuable comments on early drafts. Geoff for all his advice and practical assistance, Helen for her hard work in the background and for her vision, without which the research would not have begun. Judith for her moral support and practical help, Carol with whom the research journey began and Jill for reading early chapters. The many organizations who put out the appeal for narratives and finally all the parents who had the courage to share their experiences; without them the book could not have been written.

Some quotations and other passages are reproduced by kind permission of *The International Journal of Palliative Nursing* (Grinyer and Thomas 2001a) where they were first published.

Foreword written by George's mother Helen

Our son George was diagnosed with bone cancer when he was a first-year university student and died four years later at the age of 23. During this time I can recall very few conversations with other parents in the same situation. Perhaps this was because none of George's treatments took place in wards which specialized in the care of teenagers and young adults. Occasionally we would see other youngsters arrive or depart from ward 12 at the Royal Orthopaedic Hospital or at Outpatients, waiting for test results, for surgery, for chemotherapy, but like us their parents were usually totally and utterly focused on their own family concerns and communication was minimal.

Yet I longed to know what they were feeling, how they were managing, how was treatment going for their young adult child. I remember sitting on the ward balcony one August afternoon with an exhausted mother who knew that her son would not survive. Her farmer husband simply couldn't cope with this knowledge and left the house before they were all awake and came back late in the evening in an attempt to avoid the pain of it all. At that time we thought that George's treatment would be successful and so it seemed inconsiderate to inflict my own lesser worries on her. About 18 months later we talked briefly to another mother, a bright, cheerful woman whose daughter was waiting for a check-up and whose surgery and chemotherapy appeared to have kept her well for several years. We were waiting at the same clinic to find out what, if anything could be done about George's newly diagnosed lung metastases, an occurrence this mother must have dreaded for her own daughter. So again contact was limited by our own separate anxieties and differing circumstances.

I therefore realized quite early on in George's illness that not only would we meet very few parents in the same situation, when we did the pain of it all was likely to be too great for us to share face to face. But I desperately wanted to find out whether the problems we were encountering were common experiences. From my social work background I was sure that they were. So I did what I usually do in such circumstances and that is to look for a book. This I felt would be a much 'safer' way of digesting the information I needed – in small doses and in my own time. But I was perplexed to discover that I couldn't find any written material at all that specifically addressed the needs and life-stage problems of young adults with cancer, let alone the problems their parents might encounter. This, then, is the book that I was looking for. I hope it will be found by other parents who, like me, are trying to work out how much life stage affects their young adult child's approach to a cancer diagnosis and the significance of this for their role as parents. I think, also, that it is important to stress that I was looking for this sort of information early on in George's illness, when there was a strong possibility of a cure, and that the narratives we have collected clearly indicate that the difficulties of how best to provide support are common experiences whether or not the person survives the illness.

Of course it never occurred to me until after George's death that I would find myself in the position of actually being involved in producing the book I searched for when he was alive. I simply felt that either I had been too preoccupied or overwrought to find such a publication or that perhaps it was a particularly unusual way of wanting to make sense of what we were facing as a family and other parents wouldn't feel the same way. But now I know that this isn't so. Parents (and professionals) do want to read about how other families cope and whether there are common themes and inspiration as well as fear. I'm aware that this is a book looking at young adult cancer from parents' perspectives. At first this was a major concern knowing as I do that many of the dilemmas we faced when George was ill were because he felt very strongly that this was *his* cancer and not ours. However, it is also clear that most young adults with cancer need and depend on parental support and that anything that can be done to help their parents will in turn benefit the youngsters themselves.

It seemed to me at the time of George's illness that the fact that he was a young adult who had just 'flown the nest' was making what would have been an appalling situation at any age almost impossible. Every parent who has contributed to this book echoes the same themes of independence and the need for control. Anne's review of related texts and the way she has organized the narratives explains why this is so. However, cancer in a young adult is extremely rare – most of us have never met anyone in this situation until we are catapulted into it ourselves. As a result of this lack of experience we can feel that it is our own inadequacies or family dynamics or relationships that are somehow to blame for the fact that there are tensions and disagreements when all we want is harmony and a united approach. I hope therefore that reading about the difficulties other parents have encountered will ease the burden a little for those families who are struggling with the chaos of emotions as a young adult returns to physical and financial dependence while asserting their right to remain in control. I hope at least that such parents won't feel that in addition to all their other worries they are also to blame for the muddle that seems to be inevitable as adjustments and readjustments are constantly called for.

It is not only families but also health professionals who may have little or no experience of the impact of cancer in this age group and the life-stage issues involved. Of course the multi disciplinary teams in the specialist centres where the majority of the several hundred teenagers and young adults diagnosed with cancer each year are treated have accumulated an enormous amount of expertise. Even so, because of pressure of work and the overriding importance of medical treatments, staff in these centres are often acutely aware that they are not always able to adequately address the emotional needs of each individual patient and especially their family. Nor is funding and time always available to allow hard-pressed Health and Social Services staff the opportunities to reflect on their work and to share information and good practice with colleagues in their own hospitals and elsewhere. There is great variation here as in everything else and several respondents have referred to the excellent pioneering work of the Teenage Cancer Trust Units, though these units too wish that they could offer more support to parents. It was never the intention that this book should attempt to tell parents or professionals how to help a young adult with cancer. Yet, as you read the stories of these 28 (including George) young men and women, instances where medical staff got it absolutely and amazingly right for one particular individual stand out. The way the London hospice allowed Simon and his friends to be as much like other young Australians on a trip overseas as they could even though Simon was dying. The way in which George and we were given the diagnosis of his osteosarcoma both at Sheffield University and at the Royal Orthopaedic Hospital, the relief felt by Laura's mother when she was moved from a children's ward into the (then) new Teenage Cancer ward in Newcastle. There are examples as well of situations where parents and young adults were treated in ways that made them feel absolutely dreadful, for instance the treatment of Lynn's son, Simon R by intensive care nurses seemingly unaware of all he had already been through.

Away from the regional specialist centres an additional difficulty arises – the rarity of treating an 18–25-year-old with cancer in a local hospital or hospice and the associated lack of experience of the life-stage concerns affecting this particular age group. It is in this more local setting, when all treatment options have been tried that palliative care will often take place. I know at first hand that everyone involved finds the care of a dying youngster an enormous emotional and practical challenge. Perhaps through this book doctors, social workers, professions allied to medicine and therapists will be able to add our stories to the handful of patients they may already have encountered and in this way come to understand more about them – and their families. An increased awareness of their need for normality, for hope and for control won't make their care any less of a challenge but will hopefully serve to provide some sort of framework in which staff can locate their practice.

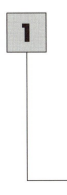

1 The impact of illness on family life

Introduction

Through narratives written by parents who have travelled on the cancer journey with a young adult son or daughter this book seeks to describe and understand the particular problems created by life-threatening illness during young adulthood. The life, illness and death of George inspired this book and each chapter begins with George's story as recollected by his mother, Helen, thus his story acts as a thread which runs through the whole book. The chapters each focus on different themes raised first through George's story; the issues are then explored further through extracts from the narratives.

Before turning to the stories written by the parents, this first chapter places in context some of the issues raised in the main body of the book by drawing on relevant research and writing. It examines aspects of life stage as they apply to adolescents and young adults and considers how illness at this time affects a family. It also deals with issues relating to the management of illness in young adults within the family situation, the different responses of mothers and fathers, the effect of illness on brothers and sisters and the financial impact on the family. It then discusses recent changes in UK Government policy as they apply to cancer and considers how an understanding of some of the issues raised in the book may contribute to the wider improvement of cancer services. Finally, the chapter presents an account of the way in which the research was undertaken, how the narratives were collected from parents and how the book is organized.

It is not the claim of this book that the death or life-threatening illness of a child at this age is a greater tragedy than at any other age or life stage, rather that there are particular problems to be faced in young adulthood in addition to the management of the illness. Although each chapter is based on a particular issue, there is an overarching theme of lost opportunities, unfulfilled potential and 'what ifs?' which runs through many of the narratives and appears to be characteristic of the threat to life at this time.

Before turning to the literature, the final word in this introduction is from one of the respondents whose daughter, Sara, died. As she so eloquently says:

> Is there a less heartbreaking time for a child to die? I doubt it. Any age is devastating for a parent. When your children grow up, you feel so much relief that they have not succumbed to a childhood disease or drowned or had some other accident: you congratulate yourself that you have brought them through to adulthood relatively unscathed. Perhaps a young dying child lacks the imagination to plan the rest of her/his life in detail, but a young adult has so many expectations of life, the life they have only lived in part. I ached for her loss. I ached for myself, for the realisation that she would not give me the grandchildren she had wanted for me. That I would not see her in a bridal gown.
>
> (Carol)

The effect on the family of life-threatening illness in a child

The majority of the respondents whose narratives are drawn on in this book relate the experiences and problems they and their family faced before, and in some cases after, the death of their son or daughter. Gordon Riches and Pam Dawson (2000) have explored the isolation and grief endured by bereaved parents and siblings when a child in the family dies, and have established that members of a family can feel uniquely alone despite being surrounded by others who share the loss. Couples find that communication with each other after the death becomes problematic and siblings speak of feelings of exclusion, guilt and resentment. The loss of a child, or of a brother or sister, Riches and Dawson suggest, threatens fundamentally the sense of self, the future and relationships. However, it is not only loss through bereavement that threatens this sense of self and security, even the families of those children who *survive* are changed forever by the experience of caring for them through a life-threatening illness. After all, the destination cannot be known when the journey begins. Just seven of the young adults whose stories are told in this book survived but as George's mother says, despite the fact that George died, she feels that she has more in common with parents whose son or daughter survived a long battle with cancer than with parents whose son or daughter died suddenly from an accident or suicide. It is then, the journey through the cancer on which this book focuses.

Professionals, friends and the wider family may all be in a position to offer valuable help during the process of bereavement (Riches and Dawson 2000). It is the contention of this book that the same applies to the journey through the illness. Yet as, thankfully, the incidence of cancer in young adults is rare, even specialist cancer nurses and other health professionals see few cases in this age group during the course of their professional practice. According to the *NHS Cancer Plan* (Department of Health 2000: 43), general practitioners will see only eight or nine new cases of cancer each year and most, if not all of these, are likely to fall outside the young adults' age range. Thus health professionals have little knowledge or experience of how the life stage of the young adult will affect their ability to manage the illness or the impact it will have on the family's dynamics.

If Riches and Dawson (2000) are correct in their claim that external support can be valuable in assisting recovery from bereavement, then it is likely that the same is true of managing the journey through the illness. One of the main aims of this book is to provide information not only to families but also to health professionals so that the acute difficulties faced by the families of young adults with cancer can be seen in context. If support of this type is not available, parents may feel that their family is dysfunctional in its response to the illness. This may result in families blaming their own dynamics rather than recognizing that in addition to the trauma that any family coping with cancer has to face, they have the additional impact of life-stage issues to contend with.

Life stage as a defining factor

There is something profoundly 'wrong' about the death of a child before its parents. While incurable illnesses claim the lives of children on a daily basis, the culture of modern Western society tends to 'push awareness of these personal tragedies to the back of our minds' (Riches and Dawson 2000: 9). Death and illness are hidden from view in a society where most acute illness and the majority of deaths are managed out of sight in hospitals and hospices. Thus as a society we are not equipped with the skills to manage serious illness and death, especially when this occurs in children or young adults. To lose a parent or a partner is traumatic, but it is a life event that is commonly experienced. However, the death of a child (at any age) runs against the natural order (Milo 1997). The same may be said of the process of life-threatening illness, it is not what parents or siblings expect to encounter in children or young adults. Nor indeed, is it what young adults themselves expect to encounter at this stage in their lives. As Brannen, Dodd, Oakley and Storey (1994: 208) observe, a commonly held view of teenagers is that they are a predominantly healthy group, and dangers such as nuclear war, pollution and threats to the environment are perceived by them as more significant than a serious illness, such as cancer.

The death of a child at any age may be considered 'unnatural' and is a tragedy. However, life-threatening illness during young adulthood may have a particularly damaging effect on family relationships and raise many problems for the management of the illness. It was the instinctive reaction of George's parents that they were faced with additional difficulties because of his age. An understanding of some of the characteristics of adolescence and young adulthood may help to place in context what happens within the family when life-threatening illness strikes this age group.

The term adopted by Apter (2001) for those aged 18–24 years is 'thresholders'. This is a highly descriptive and relevant way in which to interpret this life stage. Apter argues that there are expectations from the young people themselves, their parents, teachers and employers that after the age of 18 they will be mature and self-sufficient. The result of this expectation and consequent separation from family is that 'thresholders' become reliant to a much greater extent on friends, yet these friends do not have the stability to act as a substitute for family support. As they too are in transitional phases they tend to let each other down, argue with each other and move away in search of employment. Yet many of these young people will encounter major problems – not necessarily health-related – and because of the weakening of their family bonds may be reluctant to turn to their parents for assistance.

Apter argues that parenting a teenager is not the same as parenting a thresholder. Not only are they caught halfway between dependence and independence, they seem mature enough to have their problems under control, but in reality they are rarely mature enough to actually solve them. Despite this immaturity, Apter suggests that thresholders want to protect parents and appreciate the financial difficulties they might have.

The age group addressed in research undertaken by Brannen, Dodd, Oakley and Storey (1994) is limited to 15–17-year-olds, however, even at this younger end of the age range, they suggest that young people are moving towards greater social and economic independence. Despite the suggestion by Apter (2001) that the parenting of a teenager is qualitatively different, according to Brannen and colleagues' research findings (1994) it appears that many of the same 'threshold' issues arise. This is evidenced by their findings that a quarter of their respondents considered themselves to be 'adult', half claimed to be 'in between' and a quarter did not think of themselves as 'adult'. Thus we can see that the transitional nature of this life stage, in which childhood has not yet been fully left behind, but neither has adulthood been fully realized, is arguably characterized by a struggle for independence. This concept is of central importance as the impact of serious illness may have a profound effect on the young person's attempt at establishing independence.

The psychological models of adolescent development drawn on by Brannen and colleagues suggest that adolescence is also a time of emotional turbulence. It will come as no surprise to anyone who has lived through their children's teenage years that the parents in this study used terms such as 'moody', 'depressed' and 'ratty' to describe the behaviour of their adolescent children. In addition, these authors suggest that adolescence is a life stage when young people are expected to exhibit rudeness and rebelliousness, have no respect for their parents and refuse to listen to adult advice (1994: 27). According to Brannen and colleagues teenagers are emotional because they are at a stage where they are renegotiating relationships with their parents, and making new peer group and sexual relationships. This can weaken family bonds as young people seek the company of their peers away from parental supervision, again a manifestation of the search for independence (1994: 131).

During this period of young adulthood when independence is being sought, relationships with parents in all aspects of family life are being renegotiated. Thus, even when a young adult is well, parents' attempts to regulate behaviour can have implications for young people's health and health-related behaviour (Brannen *et al.* 1994: 126). However, when a young adult is diagnosed with an illness, the relationship with parents can be thrown into crisis. The type of illnesses referred to by these authors tend to be sore throats, cold and 'flu. If such minor illnesses as these can impact on family dynamics, how much greater must the impact be when the diagnosis is cancer?

One of the basic principles of Parsons's sick role theory (1951) is that the ill person is exempt from normal roles and responsibilities and has the right to be cared for by others. As Parsons says, 'Illness is predominantly a withdrawal into a dependent relation, it is asking "to be taken care of"' (1951: 285). This may be relatively unproblematic when applied to adults, but when applied to young people, accepting the sick role may restore the dependent status of childhood, a state from which there is not enough distance to make it acceptable (Brannen *et al.* 1994). As we have seen, young adults are struggling to establish their independent status, and may not be 'asking to be taken care of'. Indeed, they may instead resist the sick role in an attempt to retain independence. What may, however, happen is that they are forced into a situation where others must take care of them.

Given the nature of many cancers, the duration of the illness and various treatment types, much of this care will of necessity fall on the family of origin as Lynam's (1995) study of young adults with cancer shows. Despite the fact that respondents in her study were older (19–30) than many of those whose narratives are drawn on in this book, she identified the likelihood that the family of origin would be the family of care. She also suggests that the events of this life stage make the experience of illness qualitatively different from when older adults faced the same diagnosis. As she says:

> They had to make decisions about quitting, diminishing, or continuing work or taking leave of absence. The impact of the illness upon the capacity to work, or coping with diminished finances as a result of working reduced hours, became a family event. Some families, usually of origin, because of their own financial or human resources, were more readily able to provide support.
>
> (Lynam 1995: 122)

All the studies cited thus far, whether they apply to ages 15–17 (Brannen *et al.* 1994), 18–24 (Apter 2001) or 19–30 (Lynam 1995), suggest that this life stage of young adulthood is a transitional period during which family relationships are being renegotiated and independence is being sought. Thus, an enforced return to dependent status, made necessary by ill-health, has the potential to throw even the most 'stable' family into chaos. Young adults who have recently claimed their independent status may feel they can only be truly adult away from home as is shown in the following quote from Alec, a young man included in Apter's research 'You can't really be an adult when you live at home. With your Mom fussing around – well, you're just fighting for space, and can't tell whether you're really independent . . .' (Apter 2001: 73–4).

In addition, parents will have been used to having had responsibility for their children's health in infancy and childhood. Thus even though a young adult may have become independent and responsible for his or her own health, a tendency to slip back into relationships more appropriate to an earlier life stage may be difficult to resist. The effect of an unwilling return to a dependent relationship on parents is addressed through a discussion of the narrative material in Chapter 2.

It would be useful at this point to consider how responsibility for health is negotiated during adolescence. Brannen, Dodd, Oakley and Storey (1994), whose study encompasses the younger end of the age range, say that even at this early stage changes are taking place. They consider the nature of GP and hospital visits during this life stage and observe that when a parent does accompany a young adult child, it will usually be the mother, and it is more likely that a mother will accompany her daughter than her son. While a mother will see it as appropriate to accompany a daughter to seek medical advice on female health issues, their study suggests that a mother is likely to consider it inappropriate to accompany a son after the age of 16. Waiting outside the consulting room may represent a compromise and allows the young person to consult the doctor in confidence, but the mother will expect a full account after the consultation. Having been involved in health-related decisions and medical consultation throughout their children's lives, mothers in particular may find it difficult to relinquish this:

> In being excluded from the doctor's consulting room, some mothers fear missing out on important information concerning their children's state of health; either the young people do not ask the doctor the 'right questions' or they do not ask questions at all. Sometimes they fail to pass on any information gained.
>
> (Brannen *et al.* 1999: 97)

Here the situation as it relates to relatively minor illnesses is being addressed. However, when a medical consultation relates to a possible cancer diagnosis the anxieties can only be more severe. The likelihood is that the young person will still want privacy and will try to assert independence, and that the process of exclusion will be experienced by the parents (mother) as extremely stressful. There is also the question of confidentiality. Given the potential seriousness of a cancer diagnosis young adults may allow their parent(s) to accompany them to a medical consultation, but this will mean that despite being above the age of majority in some cases, they are sharing with their parents medical information which they could choose to keep private. The complexity of this situation, its management and impact on parents is the focus of Chapter 5, where the narratives demonstrate the confusion and ambiguity specific to this age group, particularly as it may cross the divide between the young person being a minor and reaching the age of majority when they are legally entitled to be the recipients of medical information.

Judgements may have to be made between 'capacity' and 'majority' during this transition period. Thornes (2001: 15) reflects that while young people over the age of 18, who have the capacity to think independently, have the right to make their own health care decisions, young people between the ages of 16 and 18 may also have this capacity. According to the Family Law Reform Act (1969) a 16-year-old is considered capable of consenting to treatment but is not able to refuse it. Thus at 16 it is possible to agree to treatment without parental consent. However, if a 16-year-old refused medical treatment, either a parent or the court could override their decision. The situation is further complicated by the 1985 Gillick principle (Thornes 2001), which requires clinicians to judge the capacity/competence of a young person even under the age of 16 and to then involve them appropriately in decisions.

The sharing of medical information when the diagnosis is cancer, may result in the need to address sensitive issues not usually discussed openly between young adults and their parents. A cancer diagnosis will frequently have implications for future fertility, thus issues of sexuality and procreation, which usually remain unaddressed between parents and adult children, may have to be confronted. Brannen and co-workers note that while some mothers will help their daughters to obtain contraception, in many families a 'blind eye' is turned to sexual activity, as the parents may prefer not to be confronted with the knowledge that their son or daughter is sexually active. The right to become sexually active without parental approval, or even knowledge, tends to accompany the independence that comes with joining the workforce and/or leaving home. Yet young adults who are diagnosed with cancer may also find that if independence, normally central to this age group, is lost then such private activity may become a family concern. Thornes (2001) suggests that parents are often surprised that their adolescent terminally-ill child has sexual feelings. If the young person is also separated by the illness from their peers as a source of information about sexual matters this can present a challenge to parents. The ways in which such delicate issues are handled by both parents and young adults in this situation are addressed through an analysis of the narratives in Chapter 4.

The effect on life trajectories

It has been established that young adults are at a transitional and emotionally turbulent life stage and that families managing any illness diagnosed in young adults will encounter significant additional problems. Given that a diagnosis of cancer amongst any age group carries its own significant psychosocial impact, when these factors are combined the result is likely to produce considerable problems for the family's management of the illness.

Costain Schou and Hewison (1999) consider the drain on 'personal resources' posed by cancer treatment and the impact of this drain on the identity and personal calendars of patients. We have already seen that identity and its construction through a bid for independence is crucial to young adults, and their personal calendars are particularly significant at this life stage when they should be moving through educational goals, beginning careers and establishing intimate relationships.

The concept of 'identity' is central to our understanding of the impact of a cancer diagnosis at this stage in life. Mishler (1999: 8) argues that the search for an all-encompassing total 'IDENTITY' (original emphasis) is not as useful as the recognition that we are all the sum of a number of 'sub-identities'. Whilst this may become increasingly true during a life where 'identity formation' is the outcome of a series of life events and relationships, at the life stage which is the focus for this book, the default identity, when other identities are lost, may be that of dependent child. Mishler's study of narratives of identity continues by observing that discontinuities and disjunctions in career paths were typical rather than unusual in his research, and he documents 'the centrality of discontinuities in adult identity formation' (1999: 13). However, changing trajectories in adult life may be experienced very differently from changes in young adulthood. As Apter says, 'the term "identity crisis" has largely been associated with adolescence' and she quotes Erikson as arguing that at no other stage of the life cycle are both the promise of finding and the threat of losing oneself so closely allied (2001: 69).

One of the particular issues related to the life stage of young adults with cancer is that of the tension between their 'life trajectory' and their 'treatment trajectory'. That is, the direction in which they 'should' be heading at this time in their life is altered by the treatment regime, which is forcing them to head in a very different direction. Thus trajectories may be in direct opposition to each other in a way that is thrown into sharp relief by the rapidity of change that would normally occur during this period in a young person's life. Costain Schou and Hewison (1999) quote extensively from Rachael, a 41-year-old teacher whose holiday to America was cancelled when her treatment for breast cancer had to be extended. Rachael was clearly disappointed by this, but we may assume that age and experience would afford her the knowledge that there would be another chance to holiday in America after the treatment was over. This case provides an example of a 'discontinuity' as identified by Mishler (1999), who suggests that such disjunctions are to be expected. However, for the young adults whose treatment trajectory conflicts with their life trajectory in terms of education or career, such a set back may seem catastrophic – which indeed it may be in reality; for example, if treatment stops young adults from taking A levels, they may not be offered a place at university. If they are unable to take university exams they may not complete their degree, or if they are unable to attend job interviews they may miss out on career or employment opportunities.

Whilst, with experience, we may realize that opportunities are rarely lost for all time (for example, it is possible to attend university as a mature student), to the young person such set backs must be unendurable when coupled with concern over illness and recovery and the fact that contemporaries are likely to be moving through those life-stage goals and leaving them behind.

The interruption of the life or career trajectory at this life stage is also likely to have a profound effect on the young adult's concept of his or her own identity. While older cancer patients are likely to have a well-established identity in their professional or personal life, this is not the case for many young adults. Costain Schou and Hewison consider the primacy of the 'calendar' in Western culture and the importance of 'knowing *who* I am exactly within it' (1999: 83). The centrality of life plans is what provides a stable source of identity legitimation (Ezzy 1993 in Costain Schou and Hewison 1999). However, the treatment calendar necessitates the formation of new life plans that clash with the personal calendar of the patient and this can have a profound effect on identity. The cancer diagnosis, according to Costain Schou and Hewison causes huge disruptions in the life calendars of individuals and it seems likely that this effect is exacerbated when experienced by young adults whose life plans are likely to be both in crisis and negotiation at this life stage. The additional effect this has on identity must also be far-reaching, as this will be closely connected to the life plans that confer identity as a student or in a profession or in an intimate relationship, all of which may be lost through the cancer diagnosis. Thus, the loss of such identity-confirming activity will be exaggerated in comparison to those being given a cancer diagnosis at a point in their lives when these identities are more firmly established. As Apter (2001) says, being an adult not only means being able to do 'grown-up' things it also means having a 'grown-up' identity, but serious illness is likely to threaten both. In a table charting the effects of life-threatening illness during young adulthood, Thornes (2001) lists interference with vocational plans and difficulties and discrimination in securing employment. Such effects hinder separation from the family and arguably result in undermining identity. These issues are reflected strongly in the narrative material presented at the end of Chapter 2 where 'thwarted plans' are discussed and in Chapter 3 where the loss of 'normality', so necessary to young adults, is the focus. Again the impact on not only the young adults, but particularly on the parents is of fundamental importance in these chapters.

The gendered response to illness and its management

We have already seen that parental accompaniment for medical consultations tends to be gendered, but it seems that the process of noticing and managing illness is also approached differently by men and women, and that these differences can lead to additional stress. Brannen and co-workers (1994) note that mothers are 'highly sensitive' in noticing signs of illness in a way that fathers are not. This is unsurprising as mothers continue to bear the major responsibility for childcare. In the research carried out by these authors it is significant that one of the fathers interviewed chose not to mention that his wife had been diagnosed with cancer, and in another instance an interview with a daughter shows her father's reluctance to speak of his wife's (her mother's) cancer.

In addition to the gendered management of illness, it is also likely that mothers and fathers will respond differently in emotional terms to illness in their children and that this difference will be exacerbated when the illness is life-threatening. Although some of the young adults whose stories are told in this book survived, most died, and as Rosenblatt (2000a) says the death of a child not only changes a parent forever, it permanently alters the parents' relationship with each other. As an individual each partner has to manage the overwhelming pain that comes with the death of a child, and as a couple they must deal with how each has changed. Rosenblatt suggests that each will have become something of a stranger to themselves and to each other. The partnership can never be the same, and many relationships run into difficulties after the death of a child. There is debate about whether the divorce rate is significantly higher in such a situation, but even if the couple stays together anger, blame and grief can result in what Rosenblatt calls an 'emotional divorce'. In some couples one partner may believe that how or when the other grieves is 'wrong' and such differences can lead to conflict.

Rosenblatt also reflects on the fact that men and women grieve in different ways. A man may feel the need to be 'strong' for his partner thus holding grief at bay, but may also feel concerned about grieving too little. A woman in Rosenblatt's study said she felt sorry for men because of the societal expectations that prevent them from expressing their feelings. The same study also observes that women are more likely to want to talk about the death and this can lead to tensions between the couple, each irritated by the other's needs. A woman is also more likely to read about grief and feel anger if her partner does not value what she tells him about the book, or refuses to read it himself. When men do read anything relating to the illness there is more chance it will be a technical or medical text than it will be one that addresses feelings and emotional issues.

Indeed, Rosenblatt (2000b), citing several authors and through his analysis of the narratives of bereaved parents, suggests that it is more likely that partners will differ in crucial ways, than that they will react in a similar way. According to Rosenblatt such differences are gendered and reflect gendered roles in wider (American) society with women talking about emotional issues outside the marriage more than men. It is significant that out of all the narratives on which this book is based, fathers wrote only two contributions (one of these sent in an account accompanied by one from his wife). Two other narratives were sent in the name of both parents. So the overwhelming majority of responses was from mothers, even if they were also speaking on behalf of their male partners. The gender difference is therefore both addressed and manifested in this book; through the narrative material that is largely written by mothers. Although not strictly a life-stage issue, the tension between parents is also apparent in the narrative material. In Chapter 8 the difference between the responses of mothers and fathers is discussed and is a thread which runs through many of the quotations.

Illness and the family: some additional issues

The effect of serious illness on siblings

In addition to the problems created by life stage, families caring for a young adult with cancer may also have to manage a number of other issues.

A significant factor to be taken into consideration is the effect that the illness may have on siblings. Much research has been carried out on the brothers and sisters of those with a life-threatening illness. Riches and Dawson (2000) argue that siblings in this position can feel isolated and invisible. They may be sent away for care; for example if they have an infection which might be passed on. Their parents' time is taken over by medical appointments and hospital stays, and the siblings in such circumstances may come to believe that their parents are concerned only with their sick brother or sister. The sick child is the focus of attention, not only within the family but also in the wider environment, and may be in receipt of charitable gifts, holidays and other 'benefits' that can make well siblings feel marginalized or resentful.

Spinetta and co-workers (1999) have carried out a detailed study of siblings whose brother or sister has cancer, and they too document the loss of parental time and attention as being problematic. In addition, amongst many other negative effects, these authors discuss siblings' guilt that they might have caused the illness and their fears that they might also become ill. They also suggest that siblings might experience problems at school, changes in family routines and loss of family cohesion, and that there may be greater expectations that the well siblings will take on additional household responsibilities.

Walter (1999: 87) cites a North American study of adolescent sibling bereavement in which 36 per cent of those siblings interviewed expressed 'blame, guilt or shame' about what they perceived as their failure to help their dying sibling or to prevent their death. The fatalities in this study were largely sudden deaths from accidents, suicide or murder however, thus some of the issues are different from those faced when the death is the result of a protracted illness.

Understandably, much of the research hitherto collected in this field has focused on the difficulties from the siblings' viewpoint. In Chapter 6 an analysis of the narratives examines the issue from the parents' perspective, and looks instead at the problems and tensions faced by parents when having to divide their time and attention during the course of the illness between a sick child and other well children.

Finance

Much is known already about the financial impact of having a chronically ill or disabled child. The vast majority of sick children are cared for at home (98 per cent) (Bone and Meltzer 1989) by parents who are less likely to be in paid employment than other parents (Bennett and Abrahams 1994). Many women will give up work to care for a child, and this can have a dramatic, detrimental and lasting effect on the family's income. In addition, there are likely to be increased expenses associated with the care of a sick child (Baldwin 1985; Beresford 1995; Dobson and Middleton 1998), thus this is not a time when a reduction in family income can be sustained without causing significant difficulties. Although there are some State benefits available to families in this position, they rarely meet the costs incurred, either in terms of direct expenditure or lost income (Corden *et al.* 2001).

Corden and colleagues' publication on the financial implications of the death of a child is based on interviews with a number of families whose child had been in need of hospice care. Their findings suggest that balancing the need to be in paid work against the need the child had for their care resulted in difficult decisions for parents. They also comment on the fact that while it tended to be mothers who gave up their paid work, fathers found this stressful as they continued in employment knowing that their child's life might be limited. They could also feel marginalized and excluded from what was happening at home, again pointing to gender differences and possible tensions arising from them. If the mother had been the one trained to manage the sometimes complex medical technology, or drug regimes, fathers could feel less confident in their ability to contribute to the care. However, Corden, Sainsbury and Sloper say that fathers were needed for assistance with heavy lifting and the intimate care of teenage sons who preferred their fathers to help (in contrast to situations where the mother is the parent who usually takes greater responsibility for care).

Corden, Sainsbury and Sloper document the need for many additional expenses associated with having a sick child at home. For example:

- the increased use of gas and electricity
- the increased use of the telephone both to organize and co-ordinate care and to keep in touch while housebound
- the need for private transport and the possible need for two vehicles in the family
- additional clothing and bedding and the need for frequent use of the washing machine
- increased expenditure on food, both for convenience purposes and to tempt the sick child to eat, and the need to buy food while on hospital visits
- adapting the house for wheelchairs, and the purchase of special equipment
- additional toys, activities and holidays – many families valued chances for trips and holidays, knowing that there might not be many more opportunities
- paying for professional help

These authors also comment on claiming benefits, and suggest that many parents miss out on their entitlements as they are unaware of their availability. However, many of the examples in their study are based on children who have a long-term disability rather than an acute and sudden illness.

Thus the problems facing the parents of young adults with cancer when claiming benefit, who may be students at the time of their diagnosis, may be different. There may also be different issues involved with the sudden onset of an acute illness rather than a long-term chronic condition.

The studies discussed here are not confined to children and young people of a particular age group, nor are they confined to cancer, but many of the problems are also likely to apply to families where a young adult has cancer. Chapter 7, which focuses on financial issues, considers whether the life stage of the young adult creates additional problems to those addressed in previous studies.

Recent policy changes in cancer care

The *NHS Cancer Plan* (Department of Health 2000) aims to reform and to improve cancer-related prevention, detection, treatment and care. Its four aims (2000: 5) are set out as follows:

- To save more lives
- To ensure people with cancer get the right professional support and care as well as the best treatments
- To tackle inequalities in health that mean unskilled workers are twice as likely to die from cancer as professionals
- To build for the future through investment in the cancer workforce, through strong research and through preparation for the genetics revolution, so that the NHS never falls behind in cancer care again.

The second aim, that of ensuring that people with cancer get the right professional support and care as well as the best treatment is the one most relevant to the purpose of this book. Clearly support and specialist care are recognized within this document as central to cancer services:

> We want patients and their families to be confident that they will receive the information, support and specialist care they need to help them cope with cancer, from the time that cancer is first suspected throughout the subsequent stages of the disease.
>
> (Department of Health 2000: 13)

However, the nature of professional support must be dependent not only on an understanding of the medical factors, but also on an understanding of the psychosocial impact of a cancer diagnosis. This as we have seen already is likely to be profoundly affected by the age of the patient at the time of diagnosis.

The need to expand the care provided by hospices to young adults has been recognized, and some specialist units have already been established whilst others are in the planning stage. Whilst the support offered by such services is to be welcomed, many young adults will not be treated in hospices, thus the care they receive in the community must be based on an in-depth understanding of the kind of issues addressed in this book.

Although it is not one of the main themes in the book, a number of the respondents said that their son or daughter wished to die at home, as George did. There is not enough material on this issue in the narratives to make any comment on its generalizability; however, if young adults are to be cared for at home this has significant implications for the family and the services they need to access. We have already seen how expensive it is to care for a sick child in the home, and how problematic it may be to access benefits. Such matters must be taken into account by the *NHS Cancer Plan* if care in the community is to be a realistic and manageable prospect for families.

There is also recognition in the *NHS Cancer Plan* that some patients have had poor experiences in relation to their cancer journeys, and that this is an area that needs attention. Whilst some patients report sensitive and thoughtful communication from professionals, others are given bad news in a deeply insensitive way and are kept in the dark about their condition. The management of medical information, prognoses and involvement in treatment-related decisions, are all made more complex by the age of young adults at the time of diagnosis and throughout the duration of their illness. Yet it is perhaps significant that no specific mention is made of this age group in the *NHS Cancer Plan* – except insofar as health promotion strategies are aimed at young people.

The *NHS Cancer Plan* pledges that resources (£2 million) will be provided for additional training for the practice of palliative care by district and community-based nurses. As the document establishes, people with cancer spend much more of their time living in their own (or their parents') home than in a hospital or hospice. Thus, a fundamental part of this training could include information on the particular problems faced by young adults and their families. Given the apparent lack of information on life-stage effects in young adulthood, this book aims to contribute to professional knowledge in this area. If professionals are aware of the likely impact at this life stage, regardless of cancer type, they will be able to offer better professional support, not only to the patient, but also to the family. This is an issue that will be addressed at the end of each chapter and discussed in relationship to the narrative data.

Research methods: The collection of the narrative data

The early stages of this research were shared with Carol Thomas[1] who co-authored a paper based on the narratives (Grinyer and Thomas 2001a).

Thus the 'we' referred to in this section refers to us both as joint researchers.

The collection of such data raises for the researcher a number of dilemmas, not least that of how such a sensitive topic as the serious illness and death of a son or daughter on the threshold of adulthood can be researched. Finding out about the life-stage issues involved relied on family members sharing their experiences and this necessarily meant their engagement with painful memories and distressing events. In asking them to share their experiences, a great deal was therefore expected of parents and other family members, and every attempt was made to ensure that involvement in the research should not exacerbate emotional difficulties and cause unnecessary further distress.

The aim of the 'data collection' methods employed was that they should allow people to impart information about their experiences on their own terms and in their own time. These issues were discussed with George's parents. It was agreed that a 'narrative correspondence' method was particularly appropriate in this context (Thomas 1998, 1999a, 1999b). This method enables 'the researched' to dictate the content of the information they share with researchers to a greater degree than is possible in most other types of social research – a strength rather than a weakness in this research context.

Much of this book is based on the narrative data written by the parents of young adults with cancer. These narratives are in effect people's own 'stories'. Frank (1997) suggests that people tell stories to make sense of their suffering and that when they turn their diseases into stories they find healing. The same may be said of the parents who have written the narratives, even though it is not their own illness of which they write or speak, they are still, in Frank's terms, 'wounded storytellers'.

The telling of stories can be a powerful way in which to communicate painful illness experiences. Cicely Saunders, the hospice pioneer, argues that she has influenced people through telling patients' stories – as she says 'this is what moves people' (Walter 1994: 69). Walter asks whether, from the diversity of stories told, one meta-story can be constructed, as individuals need to find connections with the stories of others and to bring together these stories in order to communicate to a wider audience. The bringing together of these stories, even in an edited form, and the subsequent creation of a meta-story can be an effective tool in not only the lobbying for change, but also in the creation of a 'community'. This book is intended for both purposes, to lobby for change and resources, but also to reach parents who have experienced isolation in their cancer journey and to connect them to others who have travelled the same path.

The narrative correspondence method involves making a public appeal, through relevant media, to people with particular kinds of experiences to 'tell their story' either through writing their own account of events or by independently making a tape recording of their spoken account. The written documents and self-made tapes that result then become the research materials of the project (Thomas 1999a). In this case, the public appeal took the shape of a personal statement written by George's mother, which briefly outlined the loss of her own son to cancer and explained how this had led to the current research project. During late 1999/early 2000, two versions of the statement, and an appeal to various cancer organizations (included in the Appendix), invited other people with similar experiences of supporting a young adult with cancer (aged 18–25 years) to write an account for the research project or to make a self-recorded tape, if preferred. Respondents were not requested to react to particular questions, or to address specific issues. Rather, the statement was an open invitation to 'tell your story', 'focusing on the problems and issues that you and your child faced during your child's illness'. We distributed the invitation widely in newsletters of cancer charities and self-help groups; as a press release to some regional newspapers; and as a leaflet for distribution at appropriate professional and other conferences. The fact that the statement was issued by George's mother, someone with personal experience of the loss of a son to cancer, rather than by academics, we believe contributed to the credibility and success of the research. In addition to allowing people to be in control of what they disclosed, this research method also had the advantage of generating a sample of respondents (albeit a self-selected one) for a topic where no sampling frame exists and for which there are (thankfully) relatively few potential respondents in the population.

We were aware that even the most well-meaning and sensitive of researchers can cause distress, particularly when it involves asking for information from people in vulnerable situations. We were rightly reminded of this by a supportive letter from the organization Cruse Bereavement Care in response to the project's call for narratives. This organization had decided not to place the request in the *Cruse Chronicle*, and we fully respected their decision. Their decision was based in part on previous experience of research done amongst their members who then never heard any more about the outcome, and as a result felt their experiences had been 'used'. We therefore determined that our research should be inclusive of the respondents and we have kept in touch with them throughout the research process. A short article based on the main themes raised by the narratives was published in a professional journal (Grinyer and Thomas 2001a), and George's mother took this opportunity to send a copy to all contributors in order to keep them informed of the progress of the research, to ensure them that their contribution had been valuable, and to express appreciation of their involvement. We hope that by including the respondents in the research process in an ongoing way, they will have felt part of the project; indeed without their contributions this book could not have been written.

The invitation statement certainly generated interest and the researchers began to receive telephone calls, email communications and letters of enquiry from both professionals within organizations (charities, hospices, hospitals, newspapers) and individuals with directly relevant personal experience. Some health professionals also acted as mediators, for example, by drawing the invitation statement to the attention of a parent with whom they had worked. An important methodological point associated with the narrative correspondence approach is that once a 'call for narratives' enters the public domain it takes on a life of its own. The researchers have no control over how it comes to be used by others or how it is passed on by third parties. Its movement through formal and informal networks becomes complex. This means that it is not always possible to know with precision how those who eventually responded and sent narrative material to us came to find out about the research.

Typically, a parent who had experienced the illness, and usually the death, of an adult son or daughter initially made contact with one of us by telephone or email. This was to find out more about the research, to obtain reassurance that their experience was of relevance, and to clarify what was being asked of them as a potential contributor. These first contacts may also have been made, quite appropriately, to check on the authenticity of the research project and the credentials of the researchers. A written narrative would usually, but not invariably, follow. In addition, a few of the narratives arrived without any initial contact with us having been made. One telephone contact led to a guided interview being conducted in the respondent's home because this was her preferred way of telling her story (and she lived within relatively easy travelling distance from the university).

This narrative correspondence method generated accounts of 27 young adults with cancer. All but seven of these young people had died. The illness durations, treatment regimes and tumour types involved were variable: osteosarcoma, brain tumour, non-Hodgkin's lymphoma, Hodgkin's disease, rhabdomyosarcoma, testicular cancer, melanoma, kidney tumour, spinal tumour, Ewing's sarcoma, teratoma, leukaemia, choriocarcinoma and ovarian cancer. Not all of these young adults fell strictly within our 18–25 years age range: one was only 15, but his mother wished their experiences to contribute to the research. The narrative accounts mainly took the form of long letters written by parents, telling the story of the young person's struggle with the illness and the effects of this on family members and friends. They tell about what happened; who did what, and how it felt. The written materials were in different styles and modes of address. One mother, wrote her account as if in dialogue with her lost son, opting to address him in person; in a portfolio of materials she used both poetry and prose, and included photographs of her son. In other cases, more than one narrative about the individual young person was supplied; for example, a husband and wife decided to write their own independent accounts of their son's illness and death and to send these contrasting accounts to us. One father wrote an individual account, but, most of the narratives were written by mothers, although five were sent with an accompanying letter in the name of both parents, and in some cases the accounts were clearly the product of discussion between parents. Some biographical details of the contributing parents, their families and sons and daughters with cancer are included at the end of the book. It may be helpful for readers to refer to these while reading the narrative extracts.

What motivated people to respond to George's mother's invitation, to put themselves to the trouble of writing and revisit painful territory in such a generous fashion? It is clear from some initial contact discussions and from the covering notes that accompanied the narrative accounts that participants were often motivated by the belief that our research could, in some way, assist others in a similar situation. In some cases respondents also told us that writing about these difficult events in their lives had been of personal therapeutic value. They also acknowledged the paucity of information that had been available to them, and valued the chance to provide material that might help others going through a similar experience. In addition, writing about a lost daughter or son was a means, for some people, of keeping their memory alive and of paying tribute to them. Some contributions in the form of diaries and poems had been written prior to the appeal, and parents appeared to welcome the opportunity for these private documents to reach a wider audience.

The act of writing was clearly more difficult for some people than for others, both emotionally and intellectually. It was evident that some respondents were not at all familiar with expressing themselves in writing (sometimes apologizing for their grammar and style), whilst others were comfortable with this mode of expression and wrote fluently. In initial contact discussions with people, the irrelevance of individuals' capacity to spell or 'write well', was emphasized and we encouraged them simply to 'put it down in your own words'. However, it was not just unfamiliarity with writing that posed problems for contributors. The pain of re-living the experience was too much for some people who had initially made contact, thus this narrative correspondence method inevitably excludes some people. No one opted to make a self-recorded tape, the subject matter being, perhaps, too emotional for this to be contemplated.

Those parents who responded were clearly a self-selected group who may share particular characteristics that make it more likely that they would feel able to contribute to the research by writing a narrative account of their experiences, although what those characteristics might be and how our sample might differ from those who felt unable to contribute is difficult to define. However, an assumption that most respondents would come from a particular socio-economic background or share a familiarity with the genre did not appear to be borne out by the contributions. Whether or not the contributors were used to writing all the material was invaluable to the research and to our understanding of the issues, nevertheless some of the narratives are drawn on to a greater extent than others. This seems inevitable as the selection of quotations reflects the need to illustrate specific issues and some narrative material encapsulated or represented wider experience in a very powerful way.

We responded to all the contributors by sending a card in reply, thanking them. In this way it was hoped that an appreciation of the difficulty entailed in writing the narrative was demonstrated and we sought to make the respondents feel a valued part of the research process. The opportunity was also taken to remind respondents that sections of the narratives might be reproduced in publications. Not only did no one object, some respondents expressed their wish to have their story told. However, it also became clear that while some respondents had a positive desire to have their real names in any publication, others wished to remain anonymous. Thus the quotations from the narratives are a mixture of real names and pseudonyms reflecting our respect for the preferences of the authors. Perhaps surprisingly, the majority of contributors very much wanted their real names used. Rather than seeking anonymity, they particularly wanted their son or daughter's identity to be 'honoured' through the use of their own name.

Analysis

Like other qualitative research methods, narratives do not generate representative samples, numerical data and statistically generalizable findings. Rather, the purpose is to give rise to experientially based understandings of how lives are lived (and lost). Obviously the sample is self-selected and cannot therefore be assumed to be representative. However, recurring themes in the narratives, from parents representing a variety of backgrounds and illness types, suggest a commonality of experience that sheds light on a poorly researched area. In this study, the narratives associated with the illnesses of 27 young adults have been analysed cross-sectionally in the search for common themes that have a wider resonance and relevance.

The data were rigorously analysed using methods of data reduction, display and conclusion drawing (Miles and Huberman 1994). Miles and Huberman note that extended text is dispersed, poorly structured and extremely bulky, and that in order to avoid jumping to unfounded conclusions, or over-weighting a particularly dramatic passage, certain processes must be observed during analysis. To this end the data have been subjected to codification. They have been sorted and sifted in a manner that facilitates the identification of similar phrases, themes and patterns. Through the identification of commonalties and differences, and a consideration of the relationship between the variables, a set of generalizations was gradually developed to cover the consistencies discerned in the database.

For an author-researcher, the whole project, but especially the analysis of the narrative material, required sensitivity and reflexivity. By reflexivity, I mean that I have tried to be self-aware and continuously to reflect on how my own social positioning and personal experiences are being brought to bear on my research-related actions and interpretations. I am a mother and can empathize strongly with the anguish that a child's serious illness and death causes, at whatever age. In addition, I have had a long-standing friendship with George's family and knew George well. Thus at many levels the research was emotionally demanding, and I was frequently moved to tears by the narrative material.

Note

1 Much of this section on data collection is based on an earlier methodology written by Carol Thomas.

2 The loss of independence:
the impact on family dynamics

George's story

*At 19 George had just managed to escape from home and was for the
first time really enjoying the freedom and the independence of student
life. He was making a success of student life . . . he had a nice group of
friends, and he was in a hall of residence, he appeared to be happy with
his courses. And we at home enjoyed a sense of relief that George, after
his year out, had made the transition to university and appeared to feel
it was the right decision and we were very happy that he wasn't any
longer living in the family home and that he had a life where he could
suit himself more than living at home, however free and easy you are.
So to have him come back after only two terms at university for an
indefinite period of time was devastating for all of us. I suppose to some
extent we were cushioned because we were told that he would get back
in the autumn term and then we were told he'd get back at Christmas
and then we were told he would get back the following academic year.
So in a way we didn't know that when he left Sheffield in May '95 that
he would never go back and I'm very glad that none of us did know that.
But having him home again after a year of travelling and then two terms
at university back in his old bedroom was really, really hard because he
didn't want to be there and we didn't want him to be there, at least not
for the reason he was there. Control seemed to be inextricably tied up
with George's fight for independence. He used his room as a place to
escape to; he would often be in there for hours on end with his door
firmly shut, sometimes through meal times. And I found that extremely
hard because I didn't know what he was thinking, I didn't know what
he was doing, I was worried all the time that he was going to become*

suicidally depressed. And in fact once the hurly burly of chemotherapy and surgery and the initial euphoria that it was all over ended, which took about a year, he did actually fall into really quite a deep depression. And to have him, in his room shutting us out during that time was unbearable from my point of view. George knew, and on a couple of occasions acknowledged to me, that he recognised that this situation was as painful for us as it was for himself. In fact at one time he said to me 'I can't begin to imagine what you and dad must be feeling and I can't cope with that. I can only cope with myself'. So I was grateful that at times when there was tension between us or we did disagree with the way he was coping with his illness, I knew that deep down he was aware that this was a very painful place for the whole family, not just for himself. He tended to fight over small things to try to control small things. He went along with the big things, he went along with all the treatment, the protocols and recommendations. But he fought over small things like how should he deal with the mouth ulcers, should he go for a blood test, should he take steroids to boost himself through the chemo, what he was going to eat. Eating became a huge area for control. When he was going through chemotherapy on a one week on, three weeks off regime, sometimes he would go for as long as 10 days with possibly only an odd Weetabix® and a couple of bowls of custard. And I was frantic wanting to get him to eat, aware that he'd got to build himself up for the next bout of chemotherapy. But he preferred to manage the nausea by not eating. And that was something that really I feel we could have handled better . . . we should just have respected his way of doing things. But I was off work and all I really wanted to do was actually get George through his chemotherapy on time so there were no delays and get him as strong as possible between each dose for the next dose, so eating became quite a battle ground. It was over the small things really I think that he asserted independence because he had lost so much control over the big things. On the other hand with hindsight I think that George's strategy for dealing with the whole illness was . . . a way of coping that he could live with. What he did was read a lot of literature of the 'self-help' variety. He worked out for himself that the way he thought he could beat the cancer was by working on his own emotional and spiritual well being. I know that he believed that he could cure himself through meditation and through hypnotherapy, through homeopathy and through diet and general healthy living; things he came to espouse more and more, during the course of the illness. So he could allow the medics to bombard him with cyto-toxic drugs, he could allow them to operate on the tumour in his leg and the tumours in his lungs because he, George, believed that he personally held the key to his long-term survival. He went along with what the medics were doing but believed absolutely that what he was doing was really more important.

*After the diagnosis of May '95, and during the early part of '96,
particularly in the early spring and summer of '96 when George had
recovered some strength from the surgery and the chemo he was rarely
at home, well in fact only at home in order to recover from the long
weekend in Newcastle or Sheffield or London or Leeds or wherever he
had been to stay with friends. He came back usually shattered. I was
desperately worried that this was the time that he needed to be building
up his immune system but looking back it was what he needed to do
because he didn't have very long periods like this, what he really needed
to do, I guess, was to party. And in one of his diaries he looked back
on those six months between I suppose February '96 and probably
July '96 as a very happy time when he was almost a celebrity I suppose.
And when people were so pleased to see him back being the sort of joky,
cheerful, sociable self that they had remembered from pre-illness days.
And I think it was terribly important for him to do that. But in terms of
diet and rest and all the other things you need to do to build up your
immune system it was probably not sensible, but who knows what the
most important thing is anyway.*

*I think looking back over the four years of George's battle against
cancer . . . probably the first 12 months was spent trying as a family
to work out some way that we could actually deal with the situation
of . . . enabling George to be as independent as he possibly could while
living in the family home financially and physically and emotionally
dependent on us. And it was a real balancing act and very, very hard.
And we failed as many times as we succeeded. But I think it seems . . .
to be very important to recognise that the young person themselves
knows what is best for them. It might take them a long time to work it
out and I think that's why we had tension during the first weeks and the
first year. George truly didn't know what was best for himself and he
was in chaos, emotional and physical and in every other way trying to
make sense of what had happened to him. And I think he made sense of
it by following his belief that what he did mattered most. But while he
was trying to work it out, it was very, very, hard, it was hard for him, it
was hard for us. But more and more as the illness progressed I learnt to
respect George's way of doing things, it might not have been my way of
doing things, but that seemed in the end to work best.*

The struggle for independence

The life stage of young adulthood from late teens to early 20s is one
of turbulence and transition, and is characterized by attempts to gain independence from the family of origin. Such attempts are an integral part of

the process of maturing and do not of necessity denote problems within the family, although some of the attempts to break away and claim an individual identity may result in conflict. Yet, in this transitional life stage, many young people may have sought, and found, independence before becoming ill. This can pose particular problems for the family when the young person has to relinquish a newly found independence and once again be thrown back on relationships associated with childhood and dependency.

George's mother already raises several issues relating to this life stage. She shows how George's return from university, his loss of independence, coupled with his attempts to retain control which his mother found difficult, all challenged the family in ways that seem inextricably connected to the transitory phase of young adulthood. Another mother, Sue, summarizes the life-stage issues that exacerbate the problems faced by any family of a young adult dealing with life-threatening illness. Sue, was a member of a self-help group of families whose teenage and young adult children had cancer. She was therefore in a position not only to observe the problems experienced in her own family, but also to have access to a wider network of families in similar circumstances. As we see from her account of the experiences in the self-help group, the newly found independence of young adults can act as an additional problem when managing serious illness:

> Families of young adults with a terminal illness are in a catch 22 situation. On the one hand, the parents are normally saddled with the financial responsibility, the nursing and care and agony, on the other hand their 'children' are adults and autonomous. Many of the problems to be faced are no different from those of families with younger children (e.g. school), but other areas have more in common with adult groups. It is an unsettling time of life anyway. The childlike features that trigger off universal sympathy have given way to beards, spots and rings through noses, but the adult work-based network and respected place in society is not yet functional. The result is frequently a bewildering roller-coaster ride through hostile territory.
>
> (Sue)

It is this 'bewildering roller-coaster ride' that we shall be sharing with the parents whose narratives are presented here. For as Sue says, this is indeed an unsettling time of life under any circumstances.

> Psychologically we found this to be the biggest challenge. Our 'adult' children had just left the nest and were still rather wobbly, but had experienced the first period of freedom or were just trying out their wings. Their severe illness threw them back into the lap of the family and until we had all readjusted, led to power battles in not

a few cases. Trying to be supportive but letting go at the same time is typical of this age group and is a problem that should not be under-estimated.

(Sue)

The phrase 'trying to be supportive but letting go at the same time' is probably characteristic of any parent's relationship with their young adult child and is part of a process that usually heads in one direction – that of independence. However, as Sue says, young adults with cancer are thrown back into the family in a dependent state, and the power battles she speaks of are possibly inevitable. Of her personal experience with her son Alex, Sue reflects:

> So when the shattering news came that Alex had cancer, it posed us with myriad challenges. Alex was used to being his own man, living away from home, making his own decisions and was immensely proud of the fact that he didn't need our help in any way. All of this was now lost. Emotionally, the situation was complicated. We had not lived together for the previous one-and-a-half years, now we were thrown back into a family situation we thought we had outgrown. Moreover, it came with trappings reminiscent of infancy: Alex was unable to walk (the primary cancer in the tibia was large and the bone about to fracture), was altogether weak and helpless and financially totally dependent on us again. This placed the whole family under consider-able strain.

(Sue)

There are many echoes in this account of the experience of George's family. The fact that young adults, who have tasted independence, are thrown back on relationships with those who cared for them in infancy can be seen to have an unsettling effect on family relationships that, as Sue says, are emotionally complicated. This, as she observes, may result in conflict:

> Nor was the situation clear-cut. Sometimes Alex was back to being the child again, expecting us to sort out all the unpopular difficulties such as insurance and registrations, or clamouring for an ice-cream, wanting a cuddle and a kiss and generally basking in family love. But at other times – in keeping with his age and circumstances – he was the young adult who could manage perfectly well without interfering parents, thank you very much! We also kept forgetting which role we were playing or supposed to play . . . A muddle.
>
> Realising that the crux of the problem must be his loss of independ-ence, his privacy, and his dreams, quite apart from the physical and mental torment he was going through, plus the fact that it was imperat-ive for him at his stage of life to feel that he was still the boss, we tried to manage by humouring him and letting him lash out at us. But

enough is enough. Eventually I lost patience, and we simply had to battle it out.

(Sue)

It appears here that the stresses caused by Alex's attempts to retain independence coupled with his fears for the future resulted directly in conflict within the family. Young adults, who have been thrust back into the family for care, are also likely to resent that care – it is all too easily seen as interference. Alex's mother's love for him and concern for his well-being are clear throughout her narrative, but how much should she tolerate in terms of challenging behaviour? She knows he might die, and clearly wants to make his life the best it can be under the circumstances, she will also have to live with the memories of conflict if she challenges his behaviour. Accordingly a struggle emerges between what should be tolerated and accepted as the inevitable effects of an intolerable situation, and what should be deemed unacceptable under any circumstances.

Brenda recounts similar problems. Young adults with certain cancers may sometimes require the intimate physical care from their parents that they received in infancy, such as feeding and 'changing'. Such care may result in a sense of role confusion and crisis:

Keeping to schedules and times for treatments became increasingly difficult. Miles became impossible to wake up in the mornings due to increased amounts of drugs. We would wake him in time to keep an appointment only for him to fall into a deep trance-like sleep again. He was unable to dress himself or did not want any help. Often he had soiled himself during the night and woken up demoralised. With a young child, a parent can make light of such things but in our case we were always 'treading on hot coals'.

(Brenda)

Anne also reflects on the difficulty she had in attending to her son Christopher's personal needs. Though she was a doctor herself, clearly the maternal relationship and the fact that he was 20 years old affected her ability to give him the intimate care he needed and his ability to accept it:

When I was with him I could perhaps persuade him to eat but I couldn't help him to shower, in fact the loss of any small dignity he had left. The nursing staff were wonderfully supportive, hi-tech skilled people, but there was no time for what used to be basic nursing care, really looking after the personal needs of a patient. I helped as best I could when I was with him, but he hated it, and I knew it.

(Anne)

Yet Gabrielle, who also needed to give her son Steve intimate care, did not feel that his dignity was compromised. Indeed she feels that the courage with which he faced the illness allowed all those who were needed to help him on a daily basis the ability to do so without damaging his sense of self:

> The support was brilliant ... Social Services, occupational therapy, physiotherapy ... the district nurses and eventually Marie Curie nurses. Nothing was too much trouble. But this was all because of the way you faced each day with so much courage, patience and humour. You were losing so much day by day. You had lost the use of your legs. The tumour pressing on your brain stem was slowly making you lose control of your facial, neck and chest muscles. You found it increasingly hard to chew, swallow, talk, hold your head up, breathe, cough and even smile. But your smile never left your eyes ... Throughout all this you never lost your dignity as a young man. You allowed me to look after your body as I had when you were a baby. I fed you, washed you, wiped you clean but you remained in control. You never complained. You were always grateful; best of all you were loving and trusting. The greater your physical loss became the more your spiritual belief strengthened ... I was so gentle with you, just as I had been when you were a newly born infant. You were so precious so perfect. Your trust was total. I knew you would want the driver for extra morphine when you refused strawberries and ice cream. 'Sorry mum'.
>
> (Gabrielle)

Nevertheless, Gabrielle does reflect on the loss of independence. Steve had already left home and begun a career, had travelled extensively and was involved in many sporting activities. In her letters written to Steve after his death she considers independence:

> At the age of twenty you left home to share a flat ... with Nigel. I'm so glad you had your independence, Steve. We needed to be apart in order for you to grow into the fine young man that you became.
>
> (Gabrielle)

Even after he became ill Steve needed to feel independent and attempted to set up home with a friend. This was clearly an unsustainable attempt at reclaiming his independence but one that he had to be 'allowed' to try. His mother's pain at letting him try while encouraging a probably futile attempt at independence are apparent in this extract:

> I visit you with Julie for support; perhaps I can hire her to look after you when you come out of hospital. Desperate to be independent you can only talk about getting back to the flat. You have been talking to James; he would like to share a flat with you. He knows the score; his mum is a nurse. You are going to apply to Blackhorse and ask [your employer] to support your application for a flat ... You're still desperate to be independent, still driving your car sometimes but in

increasing pain. The drugs are a nightmare, so many and they are all causing different side effects.

(Gabrielle)

As his mother probably suspected, this attempt at independence was to be brief, as Steve became more seriously ill. Gabrielle remembers this conversation:

'Sit down mum. Listen to me. No more talk of independence, I have not got long now. I want to come and live with you and Richard, make it my home again. I want you to give up work and look after me until I die, it won't be long'. How right you were, three weeks and three days left to live . . .

Although he was still fighting to retain his independence, it was clear at this stage that Steve could not return to work and his flat, so he came home from hospital to be looked after by his family.

(Gabrielle)

In this case we can see that it was Steve himself who recognized that he could no longer manage without care from his family. This may have lessened the conflict within the family, as they did not have to challenge his decision. Indeed the conflict was probably lessened when his mother supported his failed attempt to get a mortgage and share a flat, even though she knew it could not succeed.

Another manifestation of recognizing the need for independence is the fear that concern will be regarded as interference. Paul had become unwell after what his mother calls a 'round the world' visit to Canada and Mexico. Thus it is clear that he had already established his independence. His mother kept a diary of her feelings during the course of Paul's illness and death from Hodgkin's disease, and we can see the conflict between her need to be reassured of his welfare and of his need not to have to account for his every movement:

So you see – this piece of writing is once again very selfish – I need to get a grip. Paul can so I must. He's gone off to York with Chris. He went on Friday and should be back tonight. No phone call as usual! Things must be OK. Mike and I are finding it hard to know how much to ask Paul. He made it clear on Thursday that we are asking him about every move he makes. It must be infuriating to someone as independent as Paul but we need to know to keep ourselves sure he's OK. I must learn to shut up!!

(Sue B)

Such is Paul's mother's concern over her handling of her anxiety that she even refers to herself as 'selfish'. Yet from an observer's viewpoint it appears quite understandable that she should feel concern whilst at the same time understanding Paul's frustration at having to account for his welfare and whereabouts. How a parent can strike an acceptable balance between concern and respect for autonomy is unclear. The fact that it seems to be a problem for many families should at least act as reassurance that it is a 'normal' problem.

A similar dilemma is recounted by Luke, who charts his son Martin's return home from university necessitated by his illness, and the difficulties he and his wife had in allowing him independence and not doing anything that might be construed as 'interfering'. They originally accepted Martin's decision to remain at university on the basis that he would be happier there, while their concern for his welfare led to a struggle with their desire to be in close contact, telephoning to see how he was and reassuring themselves.

> He has lots of friends to talk to and support him in every way, from mother confessor to graveyard humorists. The latter is a bit cringe-worthy, and we are desperate that we only have the 'phone, do not want to appear over anxious by 'phoning every few minutes, but cannot really judge his state of mind at this distance. Our instincts tell us he will be happier amongst his friends and there is benefit in the way they will support him, so we have just told him to ring when he needed a break. Suspect it is all a novelty at this stage and may wear off.
>
> (Luke)

However, Martin's attempt at independence was to be brief. While his friends were probably willing in theory to support and care for him, in practice young people at this age are unlikely to have the wherewithal to sustain such a commitment. They too are finding their own identities and independence and are ill-prepared for the responsibility. Thus Martin returned home to the care of his parents.

> Martin phoned at lunchtime with all this and suggested he would like to come home because he did not think it fair on his flatmates to expect them to look after him for six weeks. He said he would see his tutor immediately to see how to continue the course.
>
> Martin arrived, a bit scared, which is natural and possibly more so because he has left his alma mater to come home to his boring old parents – a physical step which means 'OK, let's get it over with'. Oddly enough, I think the pressure to bear up at home is even greater than in Plymouth.
>
> (Luke)

We see here that Martin not only had to suspend his degree course, he too was forced back into dependence on the family – 'boring old parents' as his father puts it suggesting a recognition of how hard this move must have been for him.

The initial response of Barbara's son, Jamie, to being told that he would have to give up his architectural studies in London and return home for treatment was a major issue for the family. The following passage shows that Jamie's parents recognized the impossibility of him remaining in London as a student relying on his friends, and rather than let him try, and fail, as in Martin's case, his parents insisted on his return. However, Jamie's need to retain his independence resulted in a conflict about where he should have his treatment and who should care for him during its course. It is also clear from this extract that there is an expectation that the 'proper' place for a young adult with serious illness is at home with parents, and that there would be some censure from those outside the family should he not return to the family home for care.

> The biggest problem that seemed to loom was that Jamie was quite convinced he could continue in London at university and still have his treatment. 'No way' we said. 'You must give up college and come home. You have to be here. We have to be the ones that take care of you. You cannot expect strangers to be at your beck and call . . . it's not fair on them . . . And for God's sake what will people think if you continue to be in London having treatment . . .
>
> (Barbara)

Jamie, too, in the end returned home for care, albeit reluctantly.

So far the attempts to retain independence – while exemplified (by chance) by young men – could apply to either males or females in this age group but Brenda reflects on a more gendered issue in her account of the problems faced when taking her son Miles to the hospital. It seems that his need to be 'macho' overrode his need for assistance and consequently caused some distress:

> Miles absolutely refused to use a wheelchair. I believe this was very much to do with this special age group. For a formerly 'macho' young chap to be suddenly needing so much help from parents must have been degrading in his eyes. As time progressed he lost the use of his legs and could only take a few painful steps with the use of crutches. Getting him to the hospital in London, often on a daily basis, became a nightmare. We learnt not even to mention the word 'wheelchair', as he would fly into a rage. My poor husband who hated driving in London traffic had to park on double yellow lines whilst I endeavoured to help Miles from the car by the hospital, whilst my husband tried to re-park often streets away. He then would tear back to the hospital and try and find us. In the meantime I would be desperately willing Miles the strength to hobble to the hospital. People would stare at us in disbelief and embarrassment but to Miles a wheelchair was for 'little kids or old people'. He would argue about using one with nurses and doctors who always had to let him have his way. I gradually came to learn that he needed to have this little bit of control over his life and it

was not just a matter of being awkward. Many times I was convinced he would lose his balance on the shiny hospital floors.

(Brenda)

Sue had a similar experience with Alex who refused to use a wheelchair that, she says, was returned unused after his death. Although Simon R used his wheelchair (reluctantly) as it was the only way he could attend football matches, his mother, Lynn, recalls how much he hated it:

> He absolutely hated using the wheelchair, Simon did not like being seen as different and made his next goal to lose the bloody thing and forced himself into discarding the wheels.
>
> (Lynn)

Again we see a potential battleground causing parents not only anxiety but also practical problems. Yet when seen in addition to all the other indignities that were to be endured, this is perhaps a very important and symbolic stand taken by these young men.

Similarly, Iris recounts how her son Matthew insisted on driving himself to hospital. Whilst it may be the case that resistance to dependency and the enforced use of a wheelchair at any other age may be resented, when coupled with the importance of preserving newly gained independence it appears that the problems are exacerbated:

> By November 1996, he was having radiotherapy to kill off any residue and often insisted on driving his own car to and from the treatments. Someone always went with him, but he stubbornly wanted to be in charge.
>
> (Iris)

While the loss of independence and the return of the young adult to the family home may be a more common theme, the fact that young adults with cancer in this age group have adult status, and the right to make decisions for themselves, may at times add to parental anxiety. This is shown in the following account where Sianne's need to carry out the normal pursuits of young adulthood were seen by her mother as threatening to her well-being. However, her mother did not try to stop her from these activities and she was active until just before her death:

> I found it terribly hard, because I wanted to protect her but at the same time give her all the encouragement I could to get out and try everything while she could. She did amazingly well, including going to Knebworth in the middle of her high-dose treatment to see her idols, Oasis, going to V97, several holidays with her friends both at home and abroad and finally managing a week in Tenerife three weeks before she died while I remained at home in a state of sheer panic!
>
> (Candy)

We can see from Candy's account that her concern whilst Sianne was away was immense. She must also have been aware that if Sianne's death was approaching, these were days when she was sacrificing the limited time they had left to spend together, and instead encouraging her to spend it enjoying herself with others.

Likewise an extract from Sue B's diary of her son Paul's activities raises many of the same issues:

> On Thursday evening, Paul's friend from London arrived and has been with us ever since. They've managed to go out boozing and visit the Molineux to watch Wolves play. Last night Paul looked very much the worse for wear – he needs a good sleep and a couple of days without beer!! His face is puffy and blotchy and he looks exhausted. Standing at a football match takes some doing if you're not well . . .
>
> He spent a super weekend in York and then felt very tired. He's been out most nights and spent a crazy hour playing in the snow with Roadie [a friend]. Just like two little 10 year olds. I think he's given his body a real battering.
>
> The bone marrow transplant involves isolation for four weeks in hospital followed by avoiding pubs, clubs, crowds, etc. The very things that have given Paul his wonderful strength. The support of those wonderful people at the Homestead [the local pub] is terrific.
>
> (Sue B)

Again we see a mother whose concern for her son's welfare is challenged by his behaviour. Yet the knowledge that activities, such as attending football matches, drinking with friends or going to concerts are the stuff of life at this age and are in some ways what make life tolerable, must override parental anxiety. This is a phenomenon that is explored in greater detail in the next chapter.

Even greater anxiety was caused when Simon (whose home was in Australia) decided to travel across the world after having been given only weeks to live. His mother's account demonstrates the pain she felt at letting him die in the way that he wanted, in the company of his close friends:

> Soon he wanted to see only his close circle, mainly Tyson and Peter. They came together to see him on the last day of his hospital stay, and we left them to talk privately. When they'd finished, they told us that they were all going to London [from Australia].
>
> I suppose it sounds bizarre, but we agreed almost at once. We didn't think through the possibilities, we just rushed to arrange it. Everyone agreed on a two-week stay. Peter's mother told us later that he came home saying, 'I've got to sell something, I need money, Simon's got cancer and we're going to London'!! I often wonder how I would

have reacted if the tables had been turned. Would I have let Simon abandon Uni. to go overseas with a terminally-ill friend, with no outside support at all? . . . All in all, it was a week of commotion preparing for the trip, and amid this Simon wanted to visit the flat that Tyson had recently moved into with a friend. The visit was a slight taste of normality; there was teenage mess, there were videos and takeaway pizzas. But his mood was very low when we picked him up. For the last few days, his voice had been no louder than a whisper, and so he found himself unable to take part in the chat. It seems odd that it mattered so much, but I wonder whether other people find this; it's the small losses that can make or break morale in a situation like Simon's.

(Helen V)

Simon's parents therefore had to cope with his diagnosis of cancer and within weeks also with his decision to spend his remaining time away from them, on the other side of the world. Had Simon been much older or much younger such an option would have been unlikely. Clearly a child would be unable to take such a journey without its parents, and an older person might already have had some of the experiences Simon was trying to cram into his remaining days. Simon's mother, Helen V, demonstrates the pain that this trip caused her:

That was the last time we saw him alive . . . It was almost exactly a week before I started to function again. Then I really knew what suffering was. I was desperate to join Simon in London; he refused quietly but insistently.

(Helen V)

Whilst Simon was in London, he attended a hospice for treatment, but was also determined to make the most of his remaining time, causing his parents, on the other side of the world, a great deal of additional anxiety:

Meanwhile Simon was keeping appointments at the hospice, and was admitted for the night on one or two occasions. But the staff would have to persuade him to stay the next morning until the consultant came; he told them he wanted to go out sightseeing.

A week went by in this way, and then we had a phone call from Nicola [staff member] at the hospice. She said they'd suggested Simon spend every night there. Simon was non-committal on the phone to me, sounding worn out – so much so that he had to stay in the hospice anyway.

(Helen V)

Simon's parents respected his wish for them to remain in Australia. It was not until his death was imminent that they began the journey to England.

They heard while en route that he had died. As in Candy's case, we cannot imagine the sacrifice they made in respecting the wishes of their dying, adult child. It seems that at no other age would such a situation have arisen.

Again we see that the young person needs to 'normalize' life, to belong to a peer group and to undertake not only the activities usual at this age, but perhaps to undertake even greater challenges. It is clear that Simon's contact with his friends and his adventures in London were crucial to his morale, but it is also clear how difficult it was for his mother to 'let go'. Nevertheless, she says that his friends were able to offer him something that she feels the family could not:

> Friends . . . they are so central to a young adult's life; and Simon was so lucky that his were loyal and brave and willing to drop everything to go with him. They gave him quality of life. They did more than we could, because of Simon's age and his need to be independent of us.
>
> (Helen V)

That Simon's friends did more than his family could have done is debatable. Certainly had he spent his last few weeks at home with them in Australia, the experience would have been very different – though whether better or worse is difficult to judge. In this account we see a contrast to that given by Barbara of her son Jamie's attempt to stay in London with his friends for his treatment rather than to come home. Perhaps this is because Simon had been given a very bleak prognosis and only had a short time to live, in which curative treatment was not an option. Nevertheless, Simon's friends – at a similar age and life stage – can hardly have been prepared to see their friend die so far from home and support. We do not have their account of the experience and can only imagine its impact.

Even when a young adult stays close to home, the resulting lifestyle choices may feel alien to the family and may present challenges. Whilst Carol S accepted her son J's 'hippy' approach to life it is clear that she sees it at least in part as an attempt to regain control over his body:

> J was himself, an unusual young man, being quite a hippy and influenced by the New Age philosophy. We, as his parents, and also his elder brother, Steve, were relatively conservative by comparison. With all this came a travelling van parked in the drive, cannabis being puffed and, sometimes, veggy burgers cooking in the kitchen at 3 am! We are so pleased that we were able to accept all those way-out habits (as they were to us at the time) with no objections whatever. I can remember J showing me a photograph of a girl's mastectomy scar covered by a tattoo. He explained that like his ear-rings, etc. it was their own doing. They were both having appalling things done to their bodies,

over which they had no control. The tattoos and rings were embellishments of their own choosing.

(Carol S)

Whilst Carol S found J's lifestyle challenging, she is pleased to be able to look back and know that she accommodated something so alien to her own experiences. She also reflects on what she calls the 'appalling' things he did to his body. However, she recognizes that this was a manifestation of him reclaiming ownership of his body, taking control of what happened to it and making it his own creation.

The next chapter addresses the issues of 'normality' in more detail, but the issue is raised here to some extent by Candy who links it to the question of independence:

Adolescence is a time when independence should be growing but a life-threatening illness means having to be a 'child' again when they should be out having fun, making their own choices and most importantly needing to act and look *like* everyone else. One of the hardest things for Sianne to cope with was the loss of her hair, especially her eyelashes and eyebrows, and the weight she put on because of the steroids.

(Candy)

The loss of hair as a problem is a recurring theme and one that is examined in the next chapter. Candy's observation that this time of life is when young people not only need to be establishing independence but also need to be acting and looking like others is important, particularly as it may at times run counter to medical advice and parental guidance. Parents may watch their young adult children do things that make their recovery less likely and their lives shorter, and be powerless to intervene.

Whilst George was enjoying periods of remission from his illness, his mother remembers her worry when he insisted on going to parties, sleeping on friends' floors in smoky atmospheres and drinking too much. These were all manifestations of the need to normalize life, reclaim independence and to cram as much living as possible into what may be a limited lifespan. Yet for his parents who feared that such activities would undermine his health even further, they caused much anxiety.

Indeed, during the last months of George's illness he decided to cycle from Land's End to John O' Groats. An achievement he needed to make, and one his parents needed to allow him to attempt. They supported him all the way, both literally and metaphorically. He did not complete the trip.[1] Here again we see an attempt to take control of his life. In this case not by flouting convention, but by setting himself a goal he had to believe he could achieve. However worried his parents were that this trip might shorten his life they realized, as did many of the other parents whose narratives we have read in this chapter, that they needed to allow him to live the remainder of his life in his own way, whilst being there in the background to pick up the pieces as and when necessary.

The use of cannabis

The medical use of cannabis has been the subject of much controversy, but the clinical observations of doctors such as Baumrucker (2001) and Carter and Rosen (2001) suggest there are health benefits, though still the topic of scientific debate, for conditions ranging from AIDS to glaucoma. And there is evidence, according to Carter and Rosen, that cannabinoids can be used for the relief of nausea and vomiting in patients being treated with chemotherapy. Several of our respondents mentioned the use of cannabis for pain relief. While this is perhaps not a life-stage issue as defined in this research, nor an issue of independence, it may be that the use of cannabis is seen to be an 'appropriate' manifestation of youth culture amongst this age group. Indeed it may be that under other circumstances the use of cannabis would be a way of establishing independence from parental mores and culture. It may arguably be a life-stage issue in that a child would be unlikely to be offered cannabis, and an older person might be more reluctant to take it.

The results of clinical trials on the medicinal use of cannabis, sanctioned by the Government, have proved more positive than doctors, patients and even cannabis campaigners had hoped (*Observer* 2001: 6). Such an outcome might lead to the eventual legalization of cannabis for medicinal use. Even so, the police might take more convincing that its use amongst this age group is not recreational. But for the parents whose stories are told here, the use of cannabis was not legal. Thus, despite the fact that cannabis may be the only effective relief available, parents who provide their sick child with it may not only find that this challenges their lifestyle, but that they are also are taking a risk of criminal charges. In Gabrielle's case it was one she was willing to take:

> you had been catheterised twice before. They came and sorted you out but it took some time and you did not get relief until about 10 pm. Poor Steve, it was driving you mad, almost worse than pain you said. I gave you an injection of diamorphine to try to relax and calm you but the only thing that seemed to offer any relief was cannabis! You had several joints that evening! What a case for the medical use of cannabis! Over the weeks cannabis has been an important drug in the battery of drugs that we have tried to ease your pain and make your last weeks bearable. I think the fact that you could smoke it over quite a long time was a factor. What relief it gave was instant and you could keep topping it up as you smoked. Most of your drugs were given

orally, you just swallowed them down quickly and waited half an hour or so for them to start to work. You were very good; you didn't over indulge. You were always mindful of the fact that this was our house and that we were taking the risk too. I have always thought that cannabis should be used to give relief medically and this was proof before my very eyes. I would quite happily have gone to prison for letting you and your friends smoke in this house, for my belief that cannabis helped you to cope not only with your physical condition but mentally and socially too.

(Gabrielle)

It appears that Gabrielle believes that cannabis was not only of medicinal use, but also helped him 'socially'. She does not elaborate on this point, but it is possible that this was a pastime to be shared with friends. Carol's daughter Sara, a desk officer at her local police station, found that cannabis was the only effective way to provide relief for her pain:

Sara faced more chemotherapy. We had read that cannabis has an anti-nausea and relaxing effect, so I procured some through a friend. I had no conscience about using an illegal drug. Anybody who feels strongly about that should spend some time with a cancer patient undergoing cytotoxic treatment. Hospitals ought to be able to prescribe it. Sara had injections and tablets for nausea costing £20 and £38 a time – *the cannabis was the only drug that provided any true or lasting relief.*

(Carol)

For Sara, working for the police, the recognition that cannabis was the only effective drug must have posed an additional dilemma, the paradox between her professional position and her health needs creating some conflict of interest.

Reflections

The testimonies in this chapter all indicate that independence was a key issue in the management of the illness. The young adults' attempts to control their lives and maintain their independence caused problems in a variety of ways for their families. If parents allowed their sons and daughters to do as they pleased, they were consumed with anxiety for their well-being. Yet if they tried to prevent them from undertaking activities that caused concern, they faced conflict. Thus it seems that parents felt constrained to accept the actions of their son or daughter, even those which might have made their recovery less likely or their physical suffering greater. Of course, such acceptance runs counter to parents' concerns to protect their child – paradoxically a tendency that is heightened by the illness.

In addition, the loss of independence resulting in intimate care can throw family relationships into crisis. Perhaps there is little that can be done to alleviate the emotional complexity and confusions that arise from such circumstances, but parents may well be reassured to know that it is commonplace.

It is not possible to make any recommendations as to the 'right' way to manage such tensions, but the indication seems to be that however hard it was at the time to 'let go', in the aftermath of the illness parents were able to reflect on the fact that at least their son or daughter lived life to the full whilst they were able. This recognition, in some cases, appears to have been a comfort after death.

There are many echoes here with George's story. Although the bids for independence may have been manifested in different ways, by travelling away from home, by being locked in the bedroom, by not eating, by having tattoos or by not using a wheelchair – they all have something in common. That is, attempts to take control of lives whose control has been threatened by illness and by medical intervention.

We also see that the life-stage issues, as documented in Chapter 1, which relate to the emotionally turbulent and transitional nature of young adulthood and the need to establish identity through independence and separation from the family, are exacerbated by the illness. Many of the manifestations of these bids for independence are documented by Brannen, Dodd, Oakley and Storey (1994) amongst young adults who are not also struggling with life-threatening illness. For example, young adults expressing feelings of powerlessness through their intake (or lack of it) of food; by attempting to live independently; by taking risks and rejecting their parents' ideas and culture. These authors observe that when such bids for independence are made, parents steer a course between care and control. This is a course that becomes even more difficult to negotiate when the young adult has cancer.

Giddens's (1991) notion of the 'pure relationship' as one that exists only as long as both parties are in receipt of 'reflexive rewards' may be useful here in understanding the tensions played out under such conditions. The central tenet of the pure relationship as it relates to young adulthood is that, in this transitional stage, parents and young adults voluntarily renegotiate their relationship. The onus is on the young person to push for independence, and it is up to the parents to foster conditions under which the relationship can change but be sustained. The hierarchical aspects of the relationship are played down and parents become more like friends. Yet the circumstances described in this chapter throw the pure relationship into crisis.

Parents are struggling between maintaining recently negotiated relationships of trust, freedom and voluntarism, and reassuming the controlling aspects of parenthood reminiscent of an earlier life stage. However, what is also apparent from the narratives is the extreme bravery of the young people who refused simply to succumb to illness, and fought quite literally for their lives. Even where conflicts have arisen, the terms in which such bids for independence are discussed suggest parental pride in the courage demonstrated by sons and daughters in such circumstances.

Note

1 George's younger brother succeeded in undertaking the cycle ride in its entirety a year after George's death. He did this both as a tribute to the brother he had lost and to raise money for the Charitable Trust set up in George's memory.

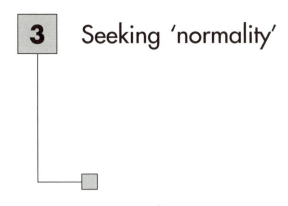

3 | Seeking 'normality'

George's story

George was a very sociable person with a very big circle of friends. At home in Lancaster most of his friends were students so they were home for long periods from their respective universities. He also still had quite a number of friends who for various reasons had not gone to university and were living locally. Friends he had made during his first two terms at Sheffield University remained in touch and one special friend from London came up by train whenever she could. His friends were desperately important to George, he needed their support, their recognition of what he was going through, and they were absolutely brilliant. There was a constant stream of cards, presents, phone calls, visits, invitations, all sorts of things just to let him know that people were thinking about him. But there were frequent periods, particularly when he was going through both lots of chemotherapy which probably amounted to a period in total I suppose of 9 months out of the 4 years, plus when he was away in Birmingham having surgery and when he had two major operations, when he was not well enough to communicate with his friends directly. And so I was acting as a go-between often on the phone, sometimes in person when people came to the door, giving George's friends information about how he was physically, how he was emotionally, and passing their good wishes on to George. And he minded this terribly because it isn't normal when you are a young man to have your mother acting as a go-between between yourself and your friends. It was even more painful when there were times I had to act as a go-between between him and his girlfriend, during the first 6 months at least of chemotherapy and surgery. He would be so poorly with mouth ulcers

*and nausea and so thin and so exhausted that I guess he probably
felt embarrassed to see her and didn't have the energy to give her the
attention that he wanted to. And so it almost felt during some of that
time that I had a closer relationship with his girlfriend, Lucy, than he
did. And living in an all-male household as I did with three sons, I valued
enormously the companionship of another woman in this situation. But it
did cause a lot of pain for George and I don't know how we could have
got round that because I was aware that his friends and his girlfriend
needed comforting and reassurance. And I felt it was important to meet
their needs as well as to meet George's needs but it was a difficult
balancing act and one that I failed at quite frequently. On the positive
side, when he was well enough to engage in the sort of activities, that
young males usually engage in, his friends were brilliant, they would
down tools and whatever he wanted to do, whether it was to play golf
when later on he was able to do that, whether it was to go to the pub,
whether it was to go to Rhodes with him as one friend did, to France as
another group did, they always made themselves available. And whatever
else was going on in their lives they were always available for whatever it
was that George needed . . .*

*At a different level he fought very hard to regain normality. After his
surgery when he had a 20 inch prosthesis in his right leg, it was very
difficult for him to even learn to walk. And so he had to work very hard
at relearning the things that mattered to him. He had been an extremely
good sportsman and it mattered to him enormously to be able to kick a
ball, to ride a bike, to swim, to play golf. And so over months he worked
and worked and within 12 months of finishing the treatment before the
secondaries appeared he could play a very decent game of golf, he could
ride a bike, and he could ride a bike long distances. I mean he could ride
30 miles in a morning without any problems and he could swim. Another
thing he did in order to try to be normal was that he registered for a
degree at Lancaster University after his first lot of lung secondaries had
been diagnosed and he had had surgery on those. And I think he truly
believed that was the end of the lung secondaries. He registered in the
autumn of '97 to begin as a student at Lancaster University. He was
thin and he was quite pale but to all intents and purposes he didn't
look different from any other young men apart from a slight limp.
This was probably 2½ years after diagnosis he registered as Lancaster
University for a philosophy degree. I absolutely know that he didn't tell
anyone that he had very recently in fact, like in August before he started
in the October, had surgery for secondary cancer. He used swimming as
a sort of therapy, as a sort of spiritual experience as well as a physical
experience. He joined the university swimming club and I don't think
anybody asked him why he had a long scar down his right leg . . . It*

*seemed to serve both those purposes because he was a very physical
person and it was one of the sports that he could do well in in spite of
the leg. He must have been an extraordinarily good swimmer in spite
of the prosthesis. But I think he was initially worried that people would
wonder why he had a scar on his chest and a scar on his leg and why he
was so skinny. But I'm pretty certain that he had decided that he was
going to tell them that he had been in a motor bike accident. That he was
not going to tell them the truth, he was going to say something that was
more macho and more normal I suppose for a young man of his age to
have experienced . . . that was one way of trying to be normal, and I
admire him enormously for it and perhaps if he had told other students
that he had got cancer, they couldn't have coped either.*

Attempts to retain normality

Adolescence and young adulthood are life stages during which belonging
to a peer group assumes great importance. In Chapter 1 we saw the significance of the tendency to spend more time with friends and away from the
family at this age as this acts as a way for young adults to establish an
identity of their own separate from that of their parents.

It appears that this need to belong can lead to a reluctance to admit
to the illness, as to do so would be to differentiate oneself from the 'norm'.
During the period when George was well enough to return to university he
left his original place of study and registered at the university in his home
town, where he told no one that he had cancer. He was also willing to
mislead his fellow students if necessary so that they would think he had
been in an accident rather than that he had cancer. So while his friends
knew, as did the students at the university he attended at the time of his
diagnosis, he went to some lengths to hide his state of health when he
began his studies again halfway through his illness. His aim was to be seen
as a 'normal' student. Normality, it appears, is central to the needs of this
age group.

This need for normality can lead to problematic situations within
families. Sue B recounts the problems created within her family because of
Paul's wish to keep his illness secret. Like George, his fear was that he
would be treated differently if people knew how ill he was. However, the
pressure put on his mother when this wish was extended to include his own
grandparents was considerable:

At last Paul gave me a few instructions, for the first time he expressed
a few feelings. He insisted that he should continue his life as normally
as possible and he didn't want everyone to know all about him in case
they treated him differently. I knew this would be difficult and tried to

explain that everyone was asking because they cared so much. However, I decided to respect his views and have requested that folks ring Marg and ask after Paul and I'd told school I'll keep in touch but please don't call. We were both very mixed up at this moment and I decided to try to head off my dear dad who I know would be calling to see how we'd got on. Too late. He began to ask questions and Paul bit his head off. He stormed up the road, swore at a driver, went in the garage and slammed the gate. I couldn't believe it when he said 'and now I've upset your son – he said he didn't want reminding'. Poor Paul and poor Dad. I explained what had happened at the hospital and Dad just sat silently. I explained Paul was cross with the world and trying to come to terms with his illness. Mom was lovely and understanding – very different from the night before when I upset her. I guess everyone's upset and mixed up. What right have we – there's nothing up with us. Paul's the one who counts.

(Sue B)

Here we see the effects on the wider family. Paul's mother is trying to manage the situation in a way which respects his wishes, but at the same time accommodate her parents' very natural desire to know what was going on. Sue B also reflects on having upset her mother the previous night. We do not have any further information on that incident, but we can see that this is a family in crisis. As Sue B says 'everyone's upset and mixed up'; but she then questions their right to be in such a state. Whilst she is correct that there is 'nothing up' with them – at least physically – there is everything 'up' with them emotionally.

Simon, at the age of 19 and diagnosed with cancer only four weeks before his death, had attempted to ignore his state of health, trying to keep up with the expectations of life as a student. As Simon's mother Helen V says:

A problem that arose from Simon's life-stage [was] . . . acknowledging that something was really wrong. It seems natural for a boy in late adolescence to cram too much into his life. I think there was a vicious circle: he felt tired and in pain, couldn't keep up with everything, got behind with some of his uni work, felt bad, etc, never stopping to say how awful he felt.

Apparently some had called him a wimp during the year because he'd been unable to keep up with them. That must have hurt him so deeply. Now he was going to tell them.

(Helen V)

It appears from this passage that Simon's attempt to be 'normal' had led to him being unwilling to seek medical advice. However, unlike George, once he had been diagnosed with cancer, he intended to tell his fellow students – possibly to account for his lack of 'normality' during the previous year when he had been struggling to keep up with them.

Gabrielle also documents the desperation of her son Steve's attempts to belong and to continue the normal activities of young adulthood.

> We shop in Watford for a designer shirt for an engagement party. You are careful to choose one that best hides your hunched broken spine. You go to the party but feel left out. You can't stand the heat of the club, can't dance, can't pull, can't even drink much, in a dying world of your own . . . You are in despair. 'Tell me how to handle this mum? I don't know what to feel. I don't know how to die'. You cried and screamed and we held you. We didn't know what to tell you to feel. Only be there with you.
>
> (Gabrielle)

It seems that Steve's attempt at 'belonging' by going to the party may have served only to exacerbate his sense of difference and the lack of normality in his life. He could do none of the 'normal' things that a young man at a party would expect to be able to do. How could his parents help him when he himself did not know what could possibly help in this situation? This confusion and concern about the most appropriate and constructive way in which to interact with a young adult child and the concern over appearance are both echoed by Charlotte:

> He was half child and half man. I was concerned about getting reassurance wrong and found it difficult at times to talk in case I accidentally made him feel worse . . . Sean needed radiotherapy to his skull and nearly refused to have it at the last minute because of hair loss. Playing in a group he was in public view. In the end he had the radiotherapy and was left with a bald patch. This was also an embarrassment because he could not go into nightclubs with friends, as he did not want to take his cap off. Arrangements were made for a hairpiece.
>
> (Charlotte)

Charlotte continues this passage by commenting that she felt that Sean was isolated by being cared for at home and that the visits from health professionals served – albeit unintentionally – to remind him of how ill he was. The 'normalization' in this case came from an old schoolteacher, paradoxically someone with whom Sean may not have had this social contact if he had not become ill:

> At home I thought Sean could be too isolated. Then, his old schoolteacher, his brother's form teacher suddenly took an interest . . . This schoolteacher was a godsend. He arranged for Sean to go out with friends for a meal. This was wonderful for my Sean – the socializing and the interest of this teacher. The teacher saw him several times.

Sean did not like seeing the district nurses too often as they reminded him (not intentionally) of how ill he was . . . Other staff came to see Sean, who knew him, and this 'normalness' really helped Sean (and me).

(Charlotte)

Charlotte uses the word 'normalness' to describe the effect that visits from friends had on both Sean and on her. Whilst much of this chapter relates to the need for the young adult to retain some semblance of normality, it is important that we recognize the importance of normality in the lives of the parents. While they are struggling with the direct results of the loss of normality for their son or daughter, their own lives have also lost that same sense of normality.

In contrast to the isolation experienced by Sean, George appears to have had much support from his friends whose availability seems to have almost been too much at times for him to cope with. During periods of better health he made the most of the chance to engage in activity with them, but when he was ill his mother needed to act as an intermediary – both with his friends and his girlfriend. This too affected the 'normality' of both his life and that of his mother, whilst she reflects on how much she valued the closeness with his girlfriend, she also recognizes that this is not 'normal'.

Despite the need for contact with his friends George's mother also says that at times he was embarrassed by his appearance and this resulted in his withdrawal. This dichotomy is also addressed in the following extract from Christine that focuses on Tony's need to continue normal activities and his concern over his hair – a problem already identified in Sean's story.

Because I think at Tony's age, because it's the time in your life where it is very, very, important you know with your friends going out and like playing football and that is normal things . . . what happened to Tony, they actually gave him high dosage chemotherapy, it's like they take your stem cells out, so it was quite high dosage . . . he's already got fair hair now, but because of the treatment he has got a bald patch on his head and we have asked at the hospital and everything, but I don't know whether that'll grow again. I don't think it will now . . . So that is a major, major problem for Tony . . . a major problem and it holds him back.

(Christine)

The importance of appearance at this age cannot be overestimated. Hair loss was mentioned in the previous chapter as an issue and arises in many of the narratives as we see in the following account of Lynn's son Simon R:

So being the brave bastards we are we just got on with it, as you do and following horrendous bouts of sickness, infections, constipation, rapid weight and hair loss (love him – this was the hardest part for him – he hated losing his hair and was so offended when anyone said it suited him to be as bald as a coot). They probably thought they were being kind but they were NOT.

(Lynn)

Here we see that even in comparison with the litany of side effects of the illness and its treatment, hair loss was 'the hardest part' for Simon R. The narratives mention the loss of hair as particularly problematic. Some young men, such as Paul, initially refused invitations to parties as a result of hair loss. But on being persuaded to go found that their friends were supportive and they could still enjoy themselves.

Despite the physical manifestations of the illness – or treatment – many of the young adults establish the importance of trying to continue to undertake all the usual activities of young adulthood. This is documented by Iris whose son Matthew also attempted to continue with 'normal' life:

Mat was in hospital just five days. He had his operation on the Wednesday and was home on the Saturday. He must have been in terrible pain, but he insisted that his brother and his dad take him to the pub that same day . . . His illness never stopped him doing the things other lads of that age did. If he couldn't drive himself, he got his brother to do it for him. He loved the pub, he loved playing darts, and loved 'the crack', the life in the pub. He drank two pints and was drunk. He loved red wine.

He loved night-clubs, he loved music, he loved bowling, driving, winding up his brother (especially winding up his brother). He loved food. Steak, chicken nuggets, bacon sandwiches, beefburgers, crisps, nuts, sweets – he loved everything. He would eat peanut butter from the jar with a spoon. He would hoard biscuits, and sweets in the cupboard beside his bed. He would keep his brother awake all night, watching movies and drinking red wine. He would insist on eating steak at three in the morning, knowing full well that Nathan had to go to college the following morning, and he himself could lie in.

(Iris)

Whilst Matthew clearly continued to undertake all the pleasurable activities of young adulthood, we can also see that he perhaps did this at some cost to his family. There is no sense of criticism here, simply an observation. Perhaps this somewhat frenetic activity resembles those incidents in the previous chapter where we saw how the young adults attempted to cram as much living as possible into their remaining life.

Lynn too documents Simon R's attempt to live a 'normal' life:

Meanwhile, whilst all this crap, chemo treatment, blood tests, injections, nausea, excruciating pain, fatigue, were happening Simon was still making gigantic attempts to 'carry on as normal'. We attended the away game at Coventry, Leeds and Sheff[ield] Wednesday at home,

Saints quiz night, drinks and meals out with his friends and pub night with Big Phil. It is difficult to imagine what he was going through – he never complained, always thinking of others and their expectations of him . . . Whilst suffering from the long term side effects of his transplant, he was on buckets of medication – his oesophagus had been damaged so the tiniest morsel of food could bring on a choking fit. All the nerve endings on his feet were damaged which gave him a lot of pain and worst of all – his fingers seized up and he was unable to play his guitar, which was catastrophic. He loved playing music but unfortunately this was only one of the further blows we were to receive over the forthcoming months. But Simon managed to socialise as much as possible, attending Basingstoke Supporters Club meetings, Kuti's, a Blur Concert at Wembley (this was using his wheels but he didn't mind that as he had a good view!!) Even spending a couple of days with his University friends in Luton.

(Lynn)

It is clear how important the pursuit of such 'normal' activities were to Simon R. However, as in the previous chapter where bids for independence caused parents anxiety, the following passage shows how the pursuit of 'normal' activities can result in further ill health:

He was a bit too enthusiastic at times though, we went away to see Saints *v* Arsenal on 26th February and he felt so good he threw himself into the day which resulted in him being taken to A&E with massive damage to his knees. Bless him, he was attempting to act as normal but even that avenue of normal existence had been taken from him. By walking and standing throughout the game he had damaged his knee joints so much the fracture clinic doc diagnosed the same damage that Steve Ovett had suffered resulting in him having to retire early from athletics. We were to discover later that one of the side effects of steroids was the weakening of bone joints.

(Lynn)

Simon R's attempt to pursue 'normal' activity had resulted in serious injury. As his mother says, he had attempted to 'act as normal' but now even that option had been taken from him. On a subsequent holiday Simon R's inability to 'act as normal' was evident:

Simon found it difficult doing 'normal things' – the pool water (in our very luxurious villa) was too cold for him to take a dip, the sea was warm but too rough. He was too weak to cope with the strong currents and crashing waves – bless him. It was gut-wrenching to witness other youngsters enjoying themselves and doing all the activities that he would have done if his body had not been ravaged by this dreadful disease. However, he kept himself occupied viewing. the lovely sites (including topless bathing beauties) a visit to Valencia's football ground. This was a very hot day and I know it took a lot out of him but the determination was there, go-karting and of course lots of yummy food.

(Lynn)

How hard it must have been for Simon R to relinquish the normal holiday activities of a young man, and how difficult for his mother to be a witness to the ravages of his illness and to the normality of the other young people in contrast.

A different aspect of the search for normality is documented by Helen V who shows that even contact with a health professional of her son Simon's age group gave him some important contact with his peer group and a sense that normality was still a possibility. This account provides an interesting contrast to Sean's experience of the visits from health professionals reinforcing his patient status and the seriousness of his condition:

A small break in this dreary routine came when a student physiotherapist came and spent some time with Simon encouraging him to walk up and down the corridor, and talking to him about the paperwork he should do to defer his end of year uni exams. This contact with someone of Simon's own age, and a student, gave him a sense of connection to normal life, a sense that he'd be back in the real world before long. Though this never happened, it was so important for Simon to feel at this stage that it would. It was an approach that I only tried later – too late.

(Helen V)

The hospice where Simon was cared for on his trip to London and where he eventually died demonstrates not only the importance of 'normality', but also the sensitivity of the hospice staff in their accommodation of both Simon's need to be a 'normal' student on his travels and his need for care:

As soon as they'd got off the plane, the boys headed for the hospice (I keep calling them boys – I wish there was another term. They use the American 'guys' among themselves). I thought his visit was mainly to fill in the three or four hours before they could pick up the keys to their flat in Putney. Later though, the hospice consultant told me that Simon had been exhausted by the flight, and wanted some help. I'm still amazed at the way he was received at the hospice. It was a Saturday morning, three tall boys in black coats and with Aussie accents turned up, and yet with apparently no fuss Simon was given some boxes of liquid food supplement and was lent a wheelchair that he could use while sight-seeing. I used to be surprised at the depth of Simon's trust in the hospice staff, but writing this makes me see that it began with this first visit. I don't know much of what the boys did in London. They visited the Museum of the Moving Image, and a few shops in Oxford Street that sold the kind of games they liked to play. My brother was in Europe on business and took time off to fly to London; his impression was that they were doing 'the same kind of stuff they do in Melbourne'. He took them out to lunch at an Italian restaurant. He also mentioned Simon's trust that the hospice could supply anything he needed; at one point they were going out, wanted a taxi, and had no number to call. 'Ring the hospice', Simon apparently said, 'they'll know'.

(Helen V)

Simon's friends were willing to suspend their studies and travel with him to London. However, for some young adults this connection to 'normal' life may be made more problematic by the transitional stage of life where a career or work pattern has not yet been established, and friends are moving on, as Sue's experience from the self-help group shows:

Friends of our patients were often scattered all over the country – as they had moved on after leaving school – and could not always be at hand. And unlike older patients who would be integrated into the workplace and have a less fluctuating circle of friends, our half adults/ half children had not yet been able to establish themselves fully.

(Sue)

The above passage appears to support Apter's (2001) claim that friends in this age group tend to let each other down, either because they have moved away or because they do not possess the necessary maturity to offer support. Whilst this was not a problem encountered by George, whose friends appeared to be both available and supportive, this is not always the case. It is predictable that many friends will be geographically distant through having gone away to university or left the area for work. Geraldine, the mother of Katy who survived ovarian cancer, makes a very similar observation:

The timing was just when most of Katy's school friends had scattered around the country to various universities. She had lots of visitors in the Norfolk and Norwich [hospital] as it was the first vacation. Apart from her boyfriend, she did not have any friends visit at the Marsden. Most were simply too far away. One who was at Reading Uni. did keep promising to visit, but did not do so. This disappointed Katy more than the many who just wrote to her.

As a result of this, we found Katy was back to spending more time with us as parents socially. She had progressed through the normal preference for spending time with her peer group in her teens, but after each week in hospital Katy felt a strong need for a trip to [the] coast or country and spend time outdoors. We tried to have a trip out each weekend as a family.

(Geraldine)

Here we can see that Katy was thrown back on her parents not only for the kind of support discussed in the previous chapter, but also for social contact at a stage when her peers were, by definition, almost bound to be scattering. Her family tried to fill this gap by providing treats and outings that her mother appears to regard as a substitute for the kind of social contact she 'should' have been having.

However, it is not only friends who 'move on', Denise observes that it was Laura who left her friends behind:

> She began her first chemo on Boxing Day and from that day on she was determined to lead 'a normal life'. . . . Laura was 15 when she was diagnosed and 19½ when she died and during that time she struggled hard with her emotions and matured at an alarming rate leaving her friends behind, as they too struggled to come to terms with her illness – how she desperately fought the treatment and would not allow them to see her ill – she was such a clever actress never allowing many people to see the real Laura – in pain, vomiting, weak, high temp. mouth full of ulcers – I could go on and on.
>
> (Denise)

Laura, also determined to lead a 'normal life', was, it seems, forced to mature early as a result of her illness, thus whilst her friends may have been moving on through the orthodox goals of this life stage, Laura was maturing in a different sense. However, we still see the reluctance to allow her friends to see her through the worst manifestations of her illness.

For those young adults who recover their health sufficiently during their illness, normality may also be expressed in terms of a return to study or to work. Although Steve's return to work was to be short-lived, its importance in terms of a semblance of normality was crucial for his morale, as Gabrielle recalls:

> Work was always so important to you Steve, especially when your life was threatened. It was normality. Work was a place where customers asked you for help and didn't ask about your cancer . . . Now I am reliving the last three months, exactly 12 weeks to the day from when we knew it had really got to you and was in your bones. You were stoic. You shrugged it off and went back to work, back to normality while you could. How sensible, how mature . . . Your pain is unbearable, you can only work for short bursts, but as you say 'At least on the shop floor people treat me normally, they ask me for help'. You go on. What strength you have.
>
> (Gabrielle)

Again we see that 'maturity' is a feature of the young adult. And again we also see the quest for normality – in this instance to be seen as a professional not a patient.

An attempt to recreate 'normality' through anonymity is demonstrated by Christine's account of Tony who sought escape in the arcades of his hometown:

> But because we'd not lived here long, he liked to go on the arcades and that was the way he coped, Tony. And it was the way, nobody knew him in the amusement arcades, nobody knew him, he could mix with everybody else, nobody was going to say anything to him, so he hid himself in those arcades and I used to go with him.
>
> (Christine)

In this case we see Tony, rather than seeking out the company of his peers, was 'hiding' from them using his anonymity as protection. It is perhaps much harder to create new friendships whilst going through such an illness than it would be to maintain established ones – as George's reluctance to tell his fellow students about his illness when he started university again suggests. The evidence in this chapter and the last suggests that the majority of friends these young adults have are caring and supportive. The major problems relating to continued contact with friends seem to be embarrassment over the physical manifestations of the illness, and the likelihood of the friends' geographical distance.

Thwarted plans

As we established in Chapter 1, young adults are at a transitory stage, when many of the decisions and actions taken have life-long consequences. Thus, not only do young adults with cancer have to manage the loss of independence, normality and social disruption of their lives; they also have to face the possibility of not completing their education or training or entering the labour market – all essential aspects of 'normality'. While there may be ways to access higher education and training at a later stage, the inability to gain university entrance qualifications, to graduate, or to complete professional training, when coupled with life-threatening illness, are likely to place additional strain on all concerned.

George had to suspend his studies in Sheffield when his illness was first diagnosed; he then had to leave the university and eventually re-registered at the university in his home town. However, he was unable to complete this second attempt at his degree as his illness worsened and he was forced to abandon his studies in his second year. Such setbacks appear to be characteristic of the impact of illness at this life stage. Candy speaks of Sianne's bravery in the face of the repeated setbacks she had when trying to take her 'A' levels:

> Sianne never whined about her situation although she used to get very angry but why shouldn't she? Who wants to die when you have just

discovered how much the world has to offer? She attempted college and 'A' levels twice but was halted in her tracks twice by the disease, but whatever she was going through she was always there to support her friends in their troubles, and her compassion for others never ceased, even over her last few days in the hospice. Her smile and personality is what is imprinted on so many people's memories from tutors to friends all over the country, from all kinds of medical staff to people who only met her in the last few weeks of her life.

(Candy)

Laura too had her plans thwarted as she was prevented from fulfilling her life-long ambition of going to university:

Laura like George, fought courageously for four years achieving tremendous things – passing her driving test and owning her own car – some independence at least for a short while, gaining 9 GCSEs, 7 As and 2 A stars, 2 A levels but sadly her childhood ambition of going to uni were not to be. Laura would I know, have been a model student but we feel not only have we been robbed of a daughter, a sister, a niece, a cousin, a granddaughter . . . She too has been robbed of so many things and why? Why her? This question has never been answered and still we ask it now and will go on.

(Denise)

Here Laura's success in achieving some of the 'normal' goals of young adulthood, are contrasted with the larger losses of her life-time ambition to be a university student and of course, ultimately, the loss of her life. The loss of such promise and potential at this time of life appears particularly cruel. Both Candy and Denise have seen their daughters through to a point where their potential was clear, only to see them thwarted by illness, and both pay tribute to their daughters' courage.

Sometimes it appears that in addition to caring for their sick child, in order to maximize their chances of a return to education, parents are forced to struggle with a bureaucratic system. We can see that Donna's attempts to complete her school education were not assisted by the school:

After a recuperation period post-transplant, Donna continued with part-time education going to school when fit and having home tuition as well. She managed to sit and pass four GCSEs which was quite an achievement under the circumstances. Up to this point we had been dealing with two heads of departments in her local school – one for 1st and 2nd year and the other for 3rd and 4th year. Both had been very understanding and accommodating with Donna's needs and illness. However, over the next two years 5th and 6th years were about to change dramatically on this front.

Donna wanted to make a normal return to school on the first day of term in fifth year to outwardly appear the same as her peers hopefully building up her strength such that she would be able to attend full-time again. We had assumed that the head in question would be fully aware of her past and present situation. For those who attended school regularly there appeared to be a big transition from 4th to 5th year never mind for someone who had only attended irregularly.

Donna had to have higher biology as a precondition to being accepted for Occupational Therapy and for one reason after another the school could not accommodate this in her 6th year. We felt this was unreasonable considering her capabilities and desires but because all the places had been allocated in her absence there was no way the school could fit this in.

At this point we felt the school was being quite unreasonable and in effect jeopardising her future, and we decided to speak to the Director of Education for our area. Co-incident with this we had been staying at dad's sister's house in Edinburgh who is a primary school head teacher but also is the 'special needs co-ordinator' for the school. We were relating all of our troubles with our school to her and she pointed out that Donna should have been receiving 'special needs care' throughout all her time at school. We were quite gob smacked as we were not aware such a thing existed and here she was now in sixth year.

The end result of this was a couple of months' battle with the education authorities. As far as the 'special needs programme' they freely admitted that this existed and that we would have been entitled to it had we asked for it! I wonder how many parents know such a programme is available. Parents are already too caught up with the illness and getting from one day to the next that they do not have the time or inclination to research these things assuming that responsible authorities will provide what is ever in their power to grant. We felt really let down by the system and guilty that here we were at the end of Donna's school education – but what could she have achieved had we been aware of and utilised this 'special needs programme'?

(Donald and Annie)

Not only did Donald and Annie have to battle with a rigid system, they also discovered that Donna should have been entitled to assistance she had not received. To be told that she would have received it if they had asked for it does not appear very helpful under the circumstances. Christine too had a similar battle with her son's school when she discovered he was unable to take exams with a practical component:

But he actually did PE and he carried on doing it, because I checked with the school, and they said 'yeah they could do it'. But he got like six weeks before the exam and they turned round and they said he couldn't take his GCSE in it because they needed to see him actually physically doing it. Because nobody seems to have any guidelines, cause I asked, and they said 'yeah they could do it prior to his illness, you know assess him prior to his illness, like on his sports ability'. But for some reason, when they are taking their GCSEs they have to be timed on certain things in PE, I don't know, and he couldn't do it. But he'd studied all that time and they turned round and said 'no he can't do it'. . . he used to love doing that [football] . . . And they did that with his science exam, they did it so far and then they said 'he couldn't take his exam'. But we had home tuition coming out, you know, people teaching him, but he [only] got so far . . . I know he phoned the teacher up and the teacher said 'well who's going to do it with him?' I think they had to do like an experiment. And they said 'who's going to do it' like he was so busy, and he said 'I can't do it'. And I said 'well you're his teacher'. You know, things like that.

(Christine)

When combined with her anxiety over Tony's health, the bureaucratic struggles with the school result in his mother's desperation and frustration, both of which are all too apparent in Christine's account.

Although Timothy survived testicular cancer, and went back to university, his demoralization did not make a return to study easy; he also had to cope with the physical limitations with which he was left as a legacy of his treatment:

In the summer Timothy returned to Reading [university], picking up his studies exactly twelve months after diagnosis. That was when the roof fell in again – reactive depression had set in with a vengeance. All his friends had graduated and he could not see the point in studying if he was going to die. The University Medical Centre offered him Prozac, but no-one to talk to for three months . . . The excessive chemotherapy has affected the blood vessels in his hips and he is now, at 25, looking at a double hip replacement. He has found this very hard to take, as he can no longer play his beloved rugby.

(Jeremy and Lesley)

Although Timothy was out of university for one year only, a much shorter time than some of the other young people, he still found it difficult to return. In this case his friends had moved on during his absence and had now left. Despite his recovery from the cancer he suffered depression, and from Jeremy and Lesley's account it seems that Timothy was not convinced that he would survive. Perhaps it was a lack of belief in his future that made motivation a problem.

Tony too found it difficult to return to education after his illness and his mother's frustration at his lack of application is apparent:

He's at college but, well last year he was supposed to be going to college, but I found out he didn't go. Well he did all the way through, but he didn't do his assignments, but he's going this year. And I keep saying to him 'all your friends are ahead of you'. But he's saying 'well they didn't have cancer'. . . he just gets angry. And when he got his work, oh 'cause he's supposed to be doing his assignments now. And I said 'have you got your assignments in?' And he just goes off, you know. 'Cause I think he thinks his friends are getting on, they've all got cars and, a couple of them have got good jobs and he blames it on to the illness. But I try and say 'you can't blame it on to that like last year' 'cause I've got to be strong. I don't think he can cope much more emotionally, definitely not, and he's not as outgoing. He seems to wait for his friends to sort of like make the arrangements. Tony holds back and sort of like goes with the flow of things . . . But he had lots and lots of trouble going back to school as well, 'cause he was off school and, you know for a long time and they all knew that he had been in hospital with cancer. He found it really, really difficult to go back to school and I had so much trouble actually getting him back there because I ended up crying my eyes out one day saying 'we just can't cope' 'cause we were sort of like living it 24 hours a day. And saying 'I just can't cope with this life, we've got to get back'. 'Cause they kept saying 'you've got to get back to school'. The consultant said you know 'it's time for you to go back now' but he just couldn't go back to school, he just couldn't face it at all.

(Christine)

There are many issues raised in this extract, and Christine's desperation is obvious. She has seen Tony through the worst of his illness, but the situation in relation to his return to school is fraught with difficulties – all of them it seems a direct result of his illness and the stage at which he was struck with it. In addition to Tony's problems with returning to school-work, his friends moving on 'having cars and jobs' made him feel left out and left behind. He had also suffered the disappointment of being offered a trial for his local football team whilst he was ill and being unable to take it up. Football was his main interest and ambition, but his illness has meant that he will never now be able to play professionally.

Another lost opportunity is recounted in Sue B's account of Paul's inability to go for a job interview, which shows how hard it was for Paul to miss the chance. She speaks of his disappointment and distress at not being able to cope as he had thought he could:

On Monday one of the building agencies called to offer Paul the chance of an interview for a job, £15,000 + car. Paul decided he'd have a go – and whilst everyone was saying 'good ol' Paul' etc, I was worried. I knew it meant long hard hours, lots of driving and Paul away from home. This was a job for a fit man and I hated admitting that Paul wasn't. The interview was fixed for Thursday 10.00 am. This meant getting up at 6.30 and travelling on three trains to his destination. Thursday morning came and Paul said he couldn't do it. The disappointment he felt having to actually admit he couldn't cope was very distressing. Poor Paul. I admire him even more because of the courage it takes to admit out loud that he couldn't cope. I wanted to stay with him but had to go to work. I couldn't get him out of my head all morning and dashed off at 12.00 only to find a bright, cheerful young man playing and singing with his guitar. What resilience. How he can bounce back I'll never know.

(Sue B)

Paul 'bounced back' and Katy too still managed to complete her degree, although she found the point in her life at which she became ill even more disruptive than would have been the case had she been at a different stage. It is perhaps the parents in such circumstances who are aware of the long-term consequences of these lost opportunities and project their feeling onto their son or daughter.

The timing was at a stage in Katy's life when everything was changing. She was just starting University. I would have liked to get the initial hospital appointment before she went to Uni. The fact that she had been in pain and was waiting for an appointment added to the normal parental anxiety of off-spring leaving home for the first time. Until the problem arose I had looked at this stage very positively. Both my husband and I had been to Uni and thought Katy would enjoy the experience as well as benefit from the education. I had also been at Manchester.

This first year was very disrupted. Katy had one term at Uni, then spent the second term based at home and was in and out of hospital. Her course was Middle Eastern Studies with a high language content. She was studying Turkish and Arabic. On the suggestion of the Professor, she continued studying Turkish at home and sending in work to be marked and set aside the Arabic. She did not return to Manchester for the Summer Term except to take the Turkish exam (which she passed). Katy worked as a kitchen assistant about 30 hours per week in a residential home until the end of August.

The following year Katy was in the second year Turkish group with the friends she had made on the course in the first term and in the first year Arabic class with the freshers. The course was a four-year course with the third year normally spent abroad. The next year was when Katy's original year was abroad so she stayed in Manchester and was in the second year but also had some classes with other groups. After that Katy had her year abroad, which consisted of two five-month spells – one in Palestine and one in Turkey and then her final year in Manchester, graduating . . . in 1998.

(Geraldine)

Katy did succeed in completing her degree a year later than planned, and her mother continues this quotation by saying that she does not feel that the effect on her University study was very great. However, she acknowledges that her social life at University suffered as she effectively switched years – as Timothy did. She was no longer with the original group she had started with and though her mother does not actually say so, the problem Tony had with making new friends in a new area in the aftermath of his illness may have been an issue here. What Geraldine does say regarding friendship is:

Young people may find that their friends are less able to cope with their illness – possibly because most have little experience of serious problems at that age. Although one of my cousins who had cancer in her thirties said quite a number of her friends seemed to be avoiding her. Her comment was that it was as if they either thought she was contagious or that she might 'drop dead in front of them'.

(Geraldine)

So perhaps cancer is a problem for friends of any age to cope with. This problem may be exacerbated by age and inexperience, but as we have seen throughout the analysis so far, friends can be a tremendous support to young adults, whether as travelling companions to far-flung places, drinking buddies or just people to talk to who are outside the immediate family.

Reflections

A number of issues have been raised in this chapter, all of them relating to the loss of normality and the quest to regain it. The importance of friends appears to be crucial, but at this time of life such contact may be lost as friends move away. Where this is the case the loss is acutely experienced. However, even where friends have been available, this has presented problems for young adults with cancer who may feel too ill to socialize or may be too embarrassed about their appearance to want to be seen.

In Chapter 1 we established the importance of belonging to a peer group, and this is clearly threatened by illness. Brannen, Dodd, Oakley and Storey (1994) demonstrated the importance of establishing links outside the family at this age, and we have seen through these narratives that such links can be broken for a number of reasons. Attempts to be 'normal' can lead to an unwillingness to recognize or admit to being ill or to seek medical help, and may also result in attempts to cover the reality of the situation.

Whilst the need for 'normality' is always central at this life stage, when coupled with life-threatening illness it may be that the young adults seek 'super-normality'. This concept, it could be argued, characterizes the intense need for normality during what is a very 'abnormal' event.

It is also clear that interruptions to the life trajectory at this stage can be exceedingly disruptive. The importance of life calendars is emphasized by Costain Schou and Hewison (1999) who note that a cancer diagnosis causes huge disruptions to both life calendars and day-to-day personal calendars. The examples in this chapter of the interruption of those calendars suggest that the disruption caused by a cancer diagnosis in early adulthood arguably has an impact even more far-reaching than at any other age as the transitional stage can be damaged for all time. The transition may, indeed, never be made – into the labour market, to university, or through to graduation. We have seen in these narratives, accounts of a number of young people whose plans have been thwarted and the resulting distress as they seek to manage not only the illness, prognosis and treatment, but also the knowledge that they may never complete the transition to the next stage of adulthood.

The implications for professionals raised in this chapter, again relate in part to their need to know that life-stage issues will have to be dealt with and that the loss of 'normality' may hit harder amongst this age group. But importantly, professionals involved in the care and management of the young adult need to be aware of the crucial nature of the life calendar. We have seen some accounts in the narratives that suggest that the disruption to the transitional nature of this life stage has been exacerbated by educational establishments being rigid in their implementation of regulations. While it seems that greater flexibility would be helpful under such circumstances, it must be acknowledged that many teachers/lecturers will never encounter the scenario described due to its (thankfully) infrequent occurrence. Yet it is this very unfamiliarity that makes the management of the situation challenging to an institution that is unlikely to have the mechanisms in place to accommodate the needs of a young person with cancer. The financial implications of these issues will be discussed in Chapter 7, but at this point it is already clear that struggles with bureaucracy have led to additional stress.

If young people with cancer, whose illnesses might be protracted, are to be able to fit back into the educational system at points when their treatment trajectories allow, an understanding by professionals of the difficulties imposed by a rigid structure may result in some of the difficulties documented in this chapter being eased. The commitment in the *NHS Cancer Plan* (Department of Health 2000) to improve cancer services in the community could extend not only to the medical services, but also to a more broadly defined support structure encompassing a knowledge of such matters, and an authority to intervene, where appropriate, on behalf of the family.

Although it was not specified in the narratives, the therapeutic environment in which young adults are treated may help them to retain a sense of 'normality' if carefully designed for their age group. Thornes (2001) cites The Teenage Cancer Trust study, which establishes that young people with life-threatening or very serious illness are no different from their healthy peers and need privacy and personal space, and appropriate and private facilities for showering, drying hair and putting on make-up. In addition they need opportunities for peer interaction, especially during the evening and at weekends. Thus, a recreation area with appropriate décor and entertainment facilities, where they can make a noise without disturbing younger or older patients, can all assist in 'normalizing' the environment and minimizing the loss of normality in other respects.

Sexuality and fertility: confronting the 'taboo'

George's story

Fertility was for George a bigger issue in the weeks after diagnosis than the cancer diagnosis. He minded more the prospect of not being able to have children than he minded having the cancer diagnosis because I think he believed that he would survive the cancer diagnosis but he knew that he would almost certainly be rendered infertile through therapy. It was a very big issue and one, which I don't think he got a great deal of informed help with because for everyone else, including his parents his survival as opposed to his ability to procreate dominated all of our feelings. Fertility was really quite an important practical issue immediately after diagnosis. Because one of the first things that he had to do after the osteosarcoma was confirmed in Birmingham was to make arrangements to go for as many possible visits as he could to St. Mary's Hospital in Manchester to donate sperm which would then be frozen for use at a later date. Now his diagnosis came very close to a May Bank Holiday and I remember that he was frantic, he wanted to give as many samples as possible and I think managed to go to Manchester four times. He also minded very much wasting, as he saw it, the 10 days or so between diagnosis in Sheffield and leaving Birmingham with a cancer diagnosis 8 days later when he again thought he could have been giving sperm. I think that the manager at the lab at St. Mary's Hospital in Manchester was wonderful, I didn't ever go with him, I didn't meet her. But I know she opened the lab one time, on a Saturday morning so that he could go, and I think he got quite a lot of help and support from her. I think his father drove him to those appointments but Lucy also went with him, that was his girlfriend. And in a sense any talk about the actual mechanics of the process would I think have been between him and Lucy and not between him and ourselves, for which I think he was probably extremely grateful. I think as the treatment progressed he focused less on whether he would be able to procreate, I'm not sure how he eventually resolved it in his own mind. I do know that after his death I looked at the consent form that he'd signed when he'd given the sperm to see what he had said. And he had actually stated unequivocally that it had to be destroyed on his death and it could not be used. I found this interesting especially in the light of all the current debate about people wanting to clone their dead children which is becoming a bigger and bigger issue I think for bereaved parents. No way would George want to be cloned or even to have his sperm used to create any of his own children after his death . . . But it paled into insignificance for me in terms of the diagnosis . . . it was one more thing that had to be done. And, we just took our lead from George, we just tried to make it possible for him to go as many times as he could. But I really felt it was more to do with procreation than sexuality. It was another biological invasion of his privacy . . . No more difficult to address than the chemo and the surgery, it was just one more thing in which his life had been taken over by people with time scales that were related to the illness and to the treatment and not to his own personal plans.

In terms of sexuality, it wasn't something he discussed a great deal with me. He had a very lovely girlfriend at the time of diagnosis and after we'd picked him up from Sheffield University on the day of diagnosis we drove straight to Manchester so that he could tell her himself. At the time her father was going through very aggressive treatment at Christies Hospital for leukaemia and George had spent the previous 9 months supporting her through that. She was around a great deal in all of the early periods of treatment and diagnosis and prognosis, and was with us when he was given his diagnosis in Birmingham . . . She was taking her first year exams at the time, she brought books with her to Birmingham, stayed with us, and tried to work. She was there on the night that the consultant came to tell George and the rest of us what he was facing in terms of diagnosis and treatment . . . I was aware at that time that quite often I was actually more present in their relationship than I really should have been but I can't really see any way round that. I desperately wanted George and Lucy to stay together. I thought they were lovely together and I know that George loved her deeply and I was well aware that Lucy was being asked here to take on a bigger burden than really she could manage. She had a lot of worries about her dad, she had a lot of worries about her course. And she was trying to support George and George quite often wasn't able to acknowledge just how much she had been available for him and how much time and concern she had provided. I felt, and I don't know whether that was right or not, that *perhaps he had taken her for granted but then he was fighting for his life and how could he do otherwise? It was just a very, very difficult situation and one which inevitably ended in their relationship breaking down, I think it probably struggled and finally broke down about 18 months after George was first told he had cancer. I'm not too sure what really went on between the two of them. But I know that when a youngster like George is so ill the relationship obviously becomes much more platonic and one where the partner has to take on a caring, nurturing role. It's not an equal relationship, it's one where perhaps people are not being able to be strictly honest with one another. Maybe, I don't know, it would have ended before 18 months had George not become ill, maybe he would have met somebody else at university, who knows what would have happened . . . We didn't talk about the effect of his illness on his physical relationship with Lucy at all. It was something that I wouldn't have raised with him and he certainly didn't raise it with me.*

I do remember not long before he died we were talking about his regrets and things he'd missed and one, apart from not being able to have children, one was to actually have had a sexually fulfilling relationship again . . . I don't know what happened with Lucy, but after their relationship had broken up he hadn't felt able in the last couple of years of his life, well enough or energetic enough, to take on a new relationship. And that's something I think that he minded . . . and the break-up with Lucy was a painful thing I think for both of them. And something that he really struggled with for a long, long time but mostly by himself . . . I can tell from his diaries that it really mattered but he didn't discuss it because I think he knew how it would upset me as well. So I don't think he talked to anybody about that . . .

George's story demonstrates the significance of fertility to a young man. As his mother says, in the initial stages of his illness, soon after diagnosis, he was more concerned about his future fertility than his survival. His relationship with his girlfriend was also of central importance, though it did not survive his illness, and it is clear that he regretted not having another relationship before his death. His mother also acknowledges that she became much more involved with him and his girlfriend and their relationship than would have been the case under more normal circumstances.

Whilst George's mother says they managed to avoid confronting the mechanics of sperm donation, the narratives from other parents in this chapter indicate that they did become involved in matters of fertility. It is a matter of 'everyday' knowledge that parents and their children commonly find it difficult to talk about sexual issues, so confronting them can create confusion and embarrassment. Three-quarters of the respondents – both the parents and the children – in Brannen *et al.*'s (1994) research said that they experienced difficulties in discussing sex. It may be that once children have reached young adulthood, and are more likely to have achieved a degree of independence and distance from their parents, the more problematic such discussions can become. Yet, as we shall see, a cancer diagnosis at this age may result in the need to confront issues of both sexuality and fertility in a way that can only serve to make the illness experience even more distressing for all concerned.

The impact of illness on sexual relationships: how do parents cope?

Before turning to the problem of fertility, we shall consider the effect of the illness on the sexual relationships – or lack of them – experienced by the young adults. We can see in the following extract from Helen V that while the doctor suggested she leave and he talk to Simon on his own, Simon wanted her to remain. It is not clear if Simon knew the nature of the questions that were to come, it is also unclear what relevance they had to his medical condition, and thus he may not have been expecting them to be so intimate.

> At one stage a young registrar came into Simon's curtained space to take a more detailed history. He told Simon there would be some extra personal queries that he may prefer not to answer in front of his parents. I got up to go, but Simon shook his head wearily and said it was OK. The questions ranged from the medical to the social. He asked Simon if he drank alcohol (we were used to offering him a glass of wine, and he also drank some beer). He didn't smoke cigarettes. Yes, he'd tried marijuana a few times (I tried not to show my astonishment – I was so naive as a parent). No, he'd never had any sexual intercourse.
>
> (Helen V)

Many parents remain, intentionally or not, unaware of their adult children's experiences of sexual activity (or drug use). Yet here we see that whilst already under immense emotional stress and anxiety, both parent and child have to confront not only the illness, but also a potentially detailed account of intensely private behaviour.

Not only may the need to acknowledge a young adult's sexuality be problematic, so may the recognition of a lack of sexual experience. What Helen V learned about her son was that he had never had the experience of sexual intercourse. Under such circumstances, parents may attempt to provide their child with the opportunity of sexual fulfilment as is shown in Helen V's account:

> We talked about his lack of girlfriends, his uncertainty about approaching them. They feel just the same, I told him sadly. All these things

we'd never talked about, and now it seemed too late . . . Simon hadn't even had a girlfriend; he hadn't experienced intercourse. He and I talked about this a bit in hospital. A friend approached the local cancer information service, who have someone specialising in sexual matters and cancer. She was going to arrange a visit to a sympathetic prostitute, but Simon was never well enough. Simon and I talked quite a lot about how we should manage this – it was a huge loss for him, among many others.

(Helen V)

For a parent to arrange a visit from a prostitute must create additional emotional stress, the parents needing not only to confront their son's terminal illness but also his sexuality. However, we can also see that when an adult child has achieved a fulfilling sexual life this can be a source of pride and joy for a parent.

You had great fun with lots of friends, filled your life to the full. At last you found the girls. You always said that girls didn't fancy you but you hadn't really tried. I remember you saying shortly before your death 'At least I've had seven sexual relationships' and with a chuckle 'six actually, I lied to my mates about the first one!' You certainly made up for lost time in those last two years!

(Gabrielle)

Gabrielle clearly takes pleasure in Steve's success with girls, though his life was cut short she uses the phrase 'filled your life to the full'. In comparison with Simon who was never well enough to experience fulfilment of this kind, Steve's mother at least knows that he had experienced a sexually fulfilling relationship. However, under other circumstances, it is likely that neither of these mothers would have known specifically about their sons' relationships with women.

The unfairness of the lost potential for a fulfilling relationship is reflected on by Candy, whose daughter Sianne died:

Another thing that seems so unfair is that Sianne had met someone very special. Whether they would have stayed together who can say, but for the last six months of her life at least she was in love. He was and still is a very amazing young man. He stayed with Sianne until after she had died just stroking her head and talking to her, along with me and Sianne's older brother. Not only had she found her special one, but she was also doing so well at college and everything else she tried, as well as being a very popular and caring person. What is the point of giving someone so many gifts if they are only going to be wiped out before they can be used?

(Candy)

Again we see that some comfort is drawn from the fact that for the last six months of her life, Sianne had been in love. The contrast in the narratives so far seems to indicate that if a young adult has not experienced some of the pleasures and successes associated with this time of life this is seen as a cruel deprivation, yet when they have begun to experience them, as Sianne had done, this too is seen as a tragic loss.

Facing the end of a relationship that has been brought about by illness may also add to the trauma and distress experienced by young adults. Even in the strongest of relationships, it seems less likely that another young adult will have the resources to be able to cope with terminal illness in a partner. As both partners are likely to be studying or building a career and only just becoming independent, material and emotional resources may be unavailable, thus the relationship may break down – as George's did. The following account Iris gives of Matthew's broken engagement suggests that the illness was too much for his fiancée to manage:

> He never had much chance of doing anything with his life. He enjoyed his girlfriends and had many. He even became engaged, but broke this off when he got cancer for the second time. Cheryl wasn't coping well with his illness, and he gave her the opportunity to get out of the relationship. Before he died he admitted that he still loved her, but could see that she didn't understand about the illness.
>
> (Iris)

To have to relinquish the relationship with his fiancée, whom he admitted he still loved, in addition to facing possible death, could only have added to the anguish felt by both Matthew and his family. Whether the relationship would have been a lasting one if he had not become ill one cannot know. Similarly, had they both been 10 years older it is not possible to say whether their relationship could have survived until his death. However, Matthew's account of his fiancée not understanding about the illness suggests that its failure bore some relationship to her age.

We can see a similar account from Brenda when discussing Miles's relationship with his girlfriend. She was apparently unable to cope with the situation, and was at a stage in her life when she was probably unable to take a career break. Had she been more established in her profession, or had the young couple had their own house or flat, the outcome might have been different for their relationship. Again we cannot know that, but the pressures of illness when coupled with these other life-stage issues, can only make the situation more problematic.

> Miles's girlfriend had to move out. After some months the inevitable happened and our son's girlfriend who had been a tower of strength could no longer cope with the situation. For her own survival and to carry on the demands of her own career she had to move into a flat

with a girlfriend. She had been a wonderful help to him and us but of course had become bowed down by the caring. In some ways that became a little easier for my husband and me as we were always having to go out in the evenings or stay in our bedroom to give them a little private time together when she came home from work. Miles knew that whatever the outcome of cancer he would never be able to have a sexual relationship again. At only 23 years of age that must have been an awesome prospect. Also he knew he would always be stuck with a catheter and major bowel problems.

(Brenda)

As well as losing his girlfriend Miles also had to face the prospect that he would never again have a sexual relationship with anyone else. At this time of life relationships may be short lived under any circumstances, but young people may nevertheless assume that before too long they will meet someone else. This cannot be the case when the prognosis has such implications for intimacy. While a pre-existing relationship may survive the illness, the chances of establishing a new one are likely to be remote.

Despite this, we are told of examples when a relationship began after the onset of the illness:

Since the beginning of the year, Jody had been visiting Simon frequently and fortunately fate gave a hand and they became very close, resulting in their relationship making Simon's difficult path to the end of his short life so much easier and happier. I am content with the knowledge that Simon and Jody shared more love and closeness during their short time together than other people ever experience in a lifetime . . . Simon spent a week with Jody and her family, Rob, Maureen and Kerry during August. He was so nervous about meeting them at last, he wasn't sure how they felt about his and Jody's relationship, after all (in his words) it is not a 'normal boy/girl thing and their expectations would be too high and he didn't want them disappointed. But they also saw the something special in Simon and had a great time.

(Lynn)

While his mother expresses her pleasure in the support that this relationship gave Simon R during his illness (as did Sianne's mother), there was clearly concern that his girlfriend's parents would find the relationship problematic. This was not the case, but in the following passage which reflects on the night of Jody's 21st party celebrations, the poignancy of the occasion is clear:

It was a great party, everyone was so friendly, and Jody looked lovely, Simon was so proud of her. All his friends from Uni were there together with Big Phil of course, everything went very well including Tilly dancing herself to sleep! Simon had one last dance with Jody and we all managed to control the lumps in our throats! It was during the early hours of the morning that Armageddon struck – Simon had a massive grand-mal and we realised then that mentally he had given up as all his goals had been achieved – his main aim since the prognosis had been to get to Jody's party, this having been achieved he hadn't got the strength to carry on any more and after a very difficult journey home injected with vomit stops, he was very calm and relaxed.

(Lynn)

In another account of a relationship, which began after the diagnosis, Sue B recalls Paul's 'miraculous' meeting with an old school friend:

Then one day, a little miracle happened, Teresa, who Paul knew at Infant School, came to school to do some observation prior to a post graduate course in teacher training. She wrote Paul a letter and then came to visit. Then she came again and again . . . and she's still here.

Paul was besotted. Someone loved him just for being Paul. His illness paled into insignificance. He went out for meals, the theatre, the cinema and between September–November life appeared to be bliss. He had his down moments, his quiet moments and Jacqui was always there to listen, to advise, to coax and to care.

(Sue B)

Again we see great pleasure being taken in the happiness experienced despite the illness, so much so that Paul's illness 'paled into insignificance' in comparison with the bliss of his relationship. Sue B also says here that someone loved Paul just for being him – regardless of his illness. George's father recalls on an early visit to the oncologist that George asked him the question 'Will anybody ever love me with a metal knee?' It must be particularly hard at a time when most young people are forming romantic attachments that rely heavily on appearance to be attractive to a partner, that the physical manifestations of their illness make success in this area less likely. We have already seen in the previous chapter how important appearance can be, and while with maturity we can see that having a metal knee or experiencing hair loss should be irrelevant to finding love, it is nevertheless understandable that such a concern should arise.

Fertility

This chapter began with recognition of the importance of fertility to young adults. This is an issue that has to be confronted whatever the prognosis, as the hope must be of survival with the potential for procreation. A cancer treatment such as chemotherapy is likely to result in infertility for both women and men. Whilst the parents' overriding concern is that treatment should begin as early as is possible, regardless of the effect on fertility, as we have seen in George's mother's account, the young person may have different priorities. At least with young men the harvesting of sperm for storage and possible future use is relatively unproblematic – though the practicalities still have to be arranged and fitted into a short window of opportunity before treatment begins. However, for women the prospect is much more complicated and the harvesting of eggs for future use is a much more complex and interventionist process.

As with the problems associated with discussing sexual matters, the prospect of a parent and young adult child freely discussing sperm donation may be challenging to all parties. George's mother says that she had no discussion with him on the 'mechanics' of the process for which she says she suspects he was 'extremely grateful'. However, the prospect of sperm donation is addressed with humour in Luke's account of his son Martin's sperm donation.

> Understand his sperm were not premier league, but active enough for the serving crate on Friday. Why they cannot do the assessment and then collect the darned things on the spot escapes me. Probably something to do with the statistics of consultant events; this way they double their apparent productivity? Just wondered what would happen if we couldn't afford the rail ticket . . . Martin went off to the Middlesex to 'make his deposit in the only bank from which I shall not be asking for an overdraft'. His spirit is truly amazing. It is now six weeks since he learned about his cancer, and through a whole series of 'is this really happening to me' events – The initial scare, confirmed when they took his testicle, the histology, the notes business, abandoning his studies, leaving Plymouth, returning to Plymouth, coming home for chemotherapy, the delay over the fertility issue and then two sessions in the loo with a little pot, he still remains cheerful, even though he is frightened stiff of the chemotherapy.
>
> (Luke)

Martin survived his testicular cancer and, at the time of writing, has been cancer free for six years and is about to marry. His father now says that it remains to be seen if he is fertile, and if not whether his 'tadpoles have survived the deep freeze'. Moira's son Alasdair, did not survive the osteosarcoma in his leg, but this is her recollection of the humour with which her son addressed the issue of fertility, and her response:

> I had to be present when a chemo nurse was explaining to Alasdair the difference between infertility and impotence (he was still only 15). She said, 'Now are you sure you understand what I'm saying?' He looked at me quickly and said 'yes, it means I can have all the fun without paying the price!' Exit one very embarrassed mother!
>
> (Moira)

It seems as though in this encounter Alasdair was able to bring more equanimity to the exchange than was his mother. The notion of their teenage son – especially at the age of 15 – engaging in sexual activity is perhaps particularly challenging for mothers. But we do see that Alasdair too resorted to humour in order to manage the situation.

Again we see humour in the way Jamie and his mother dealt with the same issue:

> As part of the visit to Christie's, Jamie had to donate sperm as he would become sterile once the chemotherapy had begun. We sat at the dinner table one evening talking about the events of the day as we always did. My son has a wicked sense of humour and has a good ear for mimicking. We said how odd it was to think that in years to come he would still be able to be a father . . . to which he replied in an American accent 'Goddam it ma – how do I tell my kids they were defrosted?'
>
> (Barbara)

At the same time not all parents are able to address the issues with humour and religious and ethical concerns may make the matter more complex:

> Sean's sperm was saved and left to his partner (assuming he had one). I have spoken with the Sperm Bank and it will be destroyed. That is the law and I think it is right. (I am Roman Catholic and was a bit worried about what would happen – ethics, etc).
>
> (Charlotte)

Here we see that Charlotte had reservations about the implications of Sean's sperm being used after his death, having been harvested in the hope that he would survive and later want children with a partner he had yet to meet. Whilst she acknowledges that is both 'the law' and 'right' for Sean's sperm to be destroyed as he had died, it must still be emotionally challenging for a mother to instruct that the last vestiges of her lost son are destroyed. George too left instructions for his sperm to be destroyed, but his mother raises the issue of the cloning of dead children. This may still be in the realm of science fiction, and no parents have mentioned it in their narratives, nevertheless, with the destruction of the sperm, any hope of cloning or future reproduction is lost forever. Thus, even for those parents with strong ethical objections to such procedures, the process must still have an emotional impact.

Lynn's account of her son Simon R's response to being told he would be infertile after treatment for choriocarcinoma, shows that she felt he dealt with the prognosis better than she:

> Even when they told him he would be sterile and would lose his nuts and even maybe his life, he was so ice cool it sent shock waves of

desperation through me. I am Mrs. Stress and living with Mr Cool and Son of Mr Cool was always difficult but then it was nigh impossible . . . Simon will need to visit the sperm bank at the Princess Anne Hospital and produce sperm for them to bank as this treatment will render him infertile, oh and by the way, he will also need an Aids check just in case (!!!????).

(Lynn)

The row of exclamation marks and question marks at the end of the passage again denotes the response of a parent when confronted with an issue not usually addressed between parent and child. Lynn refers to herself as 'Mrs Stress' while she speaks of Simon R as 'Son of Mr Cool', indicating her difficulty in dealing with the situation and his apparent equanimity. In fact his 'coolness' appears to have been as difficult for her to cope with as the information he was dealing with. Perhaps she felt that in the face of his bravery, she could not allow her distress to show. In the event, Simon R was unable to produce sperm to save in a sperm bank.

While George's mother says that it was he who was the most concerned to donate sperm when she wanted the treatment to begin as soon as possible, in Timothy's case it was his parents who identified the need for sperm donation while he just wanted to get on with the treatment:

Before starting the chemotherapy Christie's arranged for him to go to a fertility clinic at St. Mary's Hospital in Manchester. Being young and at the time unattached he did not want to waste the time but just get on with the treatment. With persuasion from us and his consultant he did go to St Mary's first and hopefully he will accept it was the right decision, even though it was made by us!!

(Jeremy and Lesley)

The tension between parents and young adults in decision making is the subject of the next chapter, but here it is pre-empted by Jeremy and Lesley's account that it was their 'decision', rather than his, to donate sperm before the start of treatment. It appears that in this case Timothy was not that concerned, as a single man, about his future fertility. In contrast, Sue B tells us of the devastating effect the prospect of infertility had on Paul:

He came out and told me simply and clearly that the cancer was also in his stomach. The treatment would be chemotherapy – drugs and injections. He could possibly be infertile – this seemed to have devastated him.

(Sue B)

Paul was well aware of the implications of this diagnosis. However, Christine doesn't think that Tony has yet realized the implications for his future of his probable infertility. In the event Tony was too ill for sperm donation to be possible. His mother reflects on the problem in this passage:

I don't think he's actually old enough really to get the impact on that one 'cause he hasn't got a girlfriend. I don't think he'll realise that 'til he's about 29, or 30, when he starts thinking about settling down. I mean now he is like a young boy going out . . . and so I don't think he's realized the impact of that yet. They did try it [to take sperm] but because he was so ill and because he was so weak they couldn't actually get any out, they did try that . . . about taking the sperm out and everything. Because they wanted to get the chemotherapy started straight away . . . it was a bit of a rush but I know it was important because they actually got us an emergency ambulance from Pendlebury to Christie's and we had to be there for a certain time for them to do the tests and get the prescription, but I said 'what about the sperm?' And they went 'oh' and they didn't start the treatment for two days after. So I don't know whether it's human rights or whatever that they've got to stop the treatment to see whether they can get the sperm out of them or not, I don't know. But I felt that it was urgent that he got the chemotherapy . . . they stopped it for two days. But because he was so weak they couldn't produce . . . he still won't talk about it now.

(Christine)

Christine went on to discuss how as a single mother of a young male they both found the issue of sperm donation difficult to discuss. This was particularly the case for Tony who is now likely to be infertile, but who cannot talk about the issues with his mother. As he gets older this situation may change, but at 16 (younger than many of the respondents) he has clearly found the additional problem of fertility difficult to address – at least with his mother. Possibly if his father – estranged from his mother and living overseas – had been available to engage with him on the subject he would have found it easier. We have already seen that mother and son communications on the topic can be embarrassing but in the case of Moira and her son Alasdair it was his mother who was the embarrassed party.

The majority of respondents who mentioned the issue of fertility were the parents of young men; the only mother of a daughter to raise the subject was Katy's mother Geraldine. We have no means of knowing if there is a any significance to this gender imbalance, indeed it might be thought that young women would be more concerned about their future ability to procreate than would young men. However, it may be that recognition of the greater complexity of egg harvesting meant that it was not considered a realistic prospect and thus not addressed. However, Geraldine says

Future fertility might become a problem. At 19 Katy was not very maternal and much more concerned about getting well and getting back to uni. Specialists at the Marsden have not suggested that Katy will not be able to have children, but with only one ovary various other friends and family keep mentioning this. Katy is now married and she and her husband do want children. In due course this could emerge, and no doubt is an issue for others.

(Geraldine)

It is interesting here that it is not the hospital or specialists who have mentioned infertility, but friends and family. Is this because Katy is a young woman and recently married? In contrast to some of the young men who have been devastated at the prospect of infertility, we see in this passage that at the point of diagnosis Katy was actually more interested in getting on with her treatment and getting back to university than in her future ability to be a mother.

Reflections

We can see from the variety of different responses that fertility and sexuality have been managed and experienced in a number of ways. Some of the young men were devastated at the prospect of infertility, whilst others simply wanted to get on with treatment. Some of the parents were concerned for future fertility, whilst others saw the urgency of the treatment as a priority. There is also a discrepancy between those families where the parents found the issue difficult to address and those where it was the young adult who found it problematic. What are we to make of these contrasting accounts?

It is clear that there were different ways of responding – humour, avoidance, embarrassment by both parents and children. It is unsurprising, given the variation in families that different families found contrasting ways of dealing with the issues, and individuals within those families responded in varying ways. However, the commonality in all the accounts, whatever the response, is recognition of the sadness that the loss of fertility at such a young age brings at a life stage before most young people have had children of their own.

A similar sadness is displayed in relation to the loss of a sexual relationship. Whether the young person dies without having ever known intimacy of this kind, or whether they are in a relationship that does not survive the illness.

Again it seems that the experiences related in George's story have a resonance in many others. His relationship failed, as did many of the relationships of the other young adults whose stories we have been told, and he was also concerned about his future fertility. His parents managed the situation with skill, but his mother acknowledges that, whilst she became more involved in their relationship than would normally be the case, the extremely personal issues between George and his girlfriend in relation to sexuality remained private, as did the mechanics of the sperm donation.

The difficulties of discussing sexually related matters are documented by Brannen, Dodd, Oakley and Storey (1994). Whilst mothers were more likely than fathers to discuss issues such as reproduction and sexual behaviour, they were still in a minority. As these authors show, whilst a small minority of young people in their study confided in their parents that they had had sexual intercourse, in the main sexual activity was kept secret from parents. Yet we have seen in these narratives a need for parents to engage with information that would usually by kept private by mutual, and silent, consent. Parents become entwined in knowledge of their child's sexual experience or lack of it, both through issues of fertility and the effect on sexual relationships. Given the likelihood that such matters would have been avoided under normal conditions, the need to address these topics in the midst of the crisis of a cancer diagnosis can be experienced by all parties as immensely problematic.

The impact of cancer on sexuality and sexual relationships has been well documented. The physical manifestations of the illness and its treatment are often cited as the obvious reasons for sexual difficulties, but psychological and emotional factors can be just as damaging (Zmuda 2001a). According to Zmuda, depression and anxiety coupled with changes in body image may result in sexual dysfunction.

Chen's study of patients undergoing radiation therapy (reported by Zmuda 2001b) found that 30 per cent of patients reported that their illness had caused them to avoid sex, 38 per cent reported decreased sexual desire, 43 per cent felt less attractive and 18 per cent derived less sexual pleasure than before the illness. Chen also found that some patients feared that the resumption of a sexual relationship might precipitate a recurrence of the cancer, particularly those cancers associated with reproductive organs (Zmuda 2001b). Yet, whilst in the past few years there has been recognition that sexuality may be profoundly affected by cancer and its treatment, Zmuda (2001a) suggests that a surprising number of clinicians still do not discuss sexual difficulties with their patients and fail to recognize deep-seated indicators of severe depression, which include the inability to experience pleasure. According to Meyerowitz (2001) despite the fact that most people with cancer report a decrease in sexual function very few have discussed this with a health professional and do not know what the commonly experienced problems are in this area. That there is a lack of communication on sexuality between staff and patients would seem to be supported by Hautamaki and Nojonen (2001) whose research findings show that many patients need information about sexuality and want to discuss such matters with health professionals. However, 59 per cent of their sample of health professionals said that they discuss sexuality with less than 10 per cent of their patients. The main reason given is 'lack of education' amongst the staff.

Zmuda also argues that a partner's fears can affect a sexual relationship. There may be a concern that physical damage might result from intimacy, that they might 'catch' the cancer or be harmed by the drugs. Patients may also be so focused on their treatment regimen that they lose sight of other important aspects of their lives such as sexuality (Zmuda 2001b).

Borg argues that cancer and its subsequent treatment can have far-reaching negative consequences on sexuality. Factors related to this psychological effect include: change in self-image – particularly important to young adults; crisis related to the loss of an organ or limb; feelings of sin and shame that might stem from the belief that the cancer is retribution or punishment for past misdeeds. According to Borg, 'respect' for the patients' private lives, lack of time and specialist knowledge and fears about addressing a topic surrounded by taboo are the main reasons for it not being raised by health professionals. His recommendations for how health professionals should address such psychological effects include:

- Knowledge: health professionals must be aware of the sexual changes that result from the illness
- Empathy: health professionals should understand how diagnosis and treatment affect the whole person
- Professionalism: health professionals should recognise their own sexual issues and problems and their impact on their ability to help the patient
- Communication: health professionals should provide an opportunity for the patient to discuss their feelings.

(Borg 1999)

We can see that whilst open discussion about such issues is of fundamental importance there are barriers to this taking place satisfactorily between patient and professional. The studies discussed here relate primarily to adults older than the age group focused on in this book. If problems are experienced with the management of the situation amongst older adults it is arguable that even greater resistance might be encountered when dealing with the matter with young adults. This may be because of an age gap between patient and professional, as a result of the professional not knowing if the young adult is sexually experienced or because of the young adult not having enough confidence to broach the subject. Nevertheless, this chapter has indicated – unsurprisingly – that sex and sexuality are of fundamental importance to young adults and must therefore be the focus of health professionals' concern during care.

5 | Involvement in medical decisions: who owns the knowledge?

George's story

Throughout most of the treatment George did not have to make decisions. The only decision he really had to make was whether or not he was going to go along with the very strong recommendations from the oncologist at The Royal Orthopaedic Hospital, he really wasn't given the options to refuse . . . he was only 19, he had hardly ever been ill in his life. And he didn't really question that this was what he was facing, and nor did we . . . The whole business of medical consultation with George and our involvement was handled extraordinarily well from the start. He was seen by the university Health Centre doctor in Sheffield . . . when George turned up with a sore knee. He [the doctor] had then, I think, sat on the information over the Friday night, and had phoned the Hall of Residence early on the Saturday morning to ask the Hall of Residence Warden . . . to ask George to stay in his room and not to go out because Dr. Burton wanted to come and see him. That would have warned George that there was something amiss . . . He told George what his findings were . . . and then asked George's permission to phone us. So we got a phone call really very soon after George had been given the diagnosis. I think he just sat in his room and wandered around the campus during that time . . . I think Dr. Burton would have asked him [if he could phone us] in such a way that he couldn't say no, I mean George would be shocked. And I think Dr. Burton would have said to George, 'I would now like to ring your parents' . . . I think he was aware that this was a family matter, this was not just a matter for a student on his own, but yes he would have got George's permission, he wouldn't have done it without. But George would have given it . . . he then spent the whole of the rest of the day at the Health Centre [he] got support from the Health Centre staff who were on duty, but was also free to wander round and see his friends if he wanted to. So he had a safe place, a haven where he could go and Dr. Burton made sure he was available when we arrived. We just downed tools and drove to Sheffield . . . Geoff and I drove in more or less total silence arriving probably half past 2 in the afternoon. And we were greeted by George sitting on the grass verge outside the Health Centre looking down the road for us arriving and he looked very pale and he looked very alone but he also looked very composed and pleased to see us. He wasn't defensive . . . he was a very private person, he didn't show his affections very readily. But when we drove up and stopped he was definitely pleased to see us and keen to reassure us that everything would be all right, that he could cope, and the outcome would be good . . . He was actually able to see it from other people's points of view as well and in a way I think that set the tone for the management of the illness. George himself usually wanted to be given the medical information first on his own, but then wanted us in the consultation to be given the same information with him present . . . we left with a clear timetable of what was going to be happening over the next I suppose 6 months . . . and we were very grateful for that. And that gave us something to actually hang on to and to put our family lives around. It also gave us something concrete to do when we got home, . . . we needed to buy pyjamas and toiletries and that sort of thing. The other thing the doctor did was phone our own GP practice in Lancaster and spoke to the on-call doctor who happened to be the woman doctor in the practice who already knew us as a family . . . And I don't think he asked permission to do that . . . a lot of this happened without George questioning it and he was just very grateful that in the situation of total chaos and uncertainty, from his point of view, there were people around that knew how to do it and this had happened before to other people and the outcome could be OK.

Thinking about when conflicts with the medics occurred . . . George tended to battle over the small things, not over the big things. He . . . wanted desperately to live and he was of a scientific disposition and he accepted that if this was what was done in this particular illness then he had to go along with it. There were a few occasions where decisions had to be made. One was very early on when he went to see Professor McIllmurray at our local hospital who was going to do the chemotherapy on the instructions of the lead Hospital which was the Royal Orthopaedic in Birmingham. And George had an interview with him in which George was asked to consider becoming part of a trial . . . , not very different treatment but more intense . . . George, Geoff and I were in the consultation, Professor McIllmurray addressed all his discussion to George. Although we didn't feel like intruders, we felt that Professor

McIllmurray and George knew that it was important for us and for him that we were there, [though] we did not have a part in the decision. And George took the decision not to go on the trial ... I wanted him to go on the trial because I wanted him to do anything that could ... improve his chances of survival. But like with many decisions or all the decisions in fact that George took during the period of his treatment it turned out to be the right one because he was desperately ill on the orthodox regime of treatment. The trial would have been even more punishing than the original protocol which George really struggled with anyway ... So, as the illness progressed we learnt or I learnt that George had his own instincts about what was right for him even though they appeared to be perhaps not the decisions that we would make, they were right for George. And that was a really important lesson and I think it took at least 12 months to learn that ... Another instance where he was making big decisions on his own, was when he had had ... one lot of lung secondaries removed but about six months later new lung secondaries appeared. Just about 12 months before he died be began a period of further chemotherapy for the lung secondaries. I think it began in March '98 and finished about June '98 and that chemotherapy was again very aggressive but it had really no impact on the size of the tumour mass in his lung. And the choice that he was then facing was that he could take the risk of having this diseased right lung removed ... no more chemo was possible but it just might delay it rather than cure the spread of the cancer. That was a decision that he was left to make for himself and he had to make it within about 6 weeks from the end of the chemo which hadn't worked ... although he did not make the decision not to have the lung removed, he allowed the date to go by without a decision being made, so he made it in a sense by default. I was frantic during those 6 or 8 weeks when I was waiting every day for George to phone Professor Casson to say, 'OK I'll come down to Birmingham and have my lung removed'. George and I fell out about it and I remember a conversation in which he said to me, 'mum you would rather I died on the operating table having my lung removed, than I would die of the cancer'. And I said, 'yes George I would'. And I guess that was what it was, I was wanting to spare George the remaining 12 months of deterioration through the cancer ... at the time I felt I would prefer him to die quickly when he was still able to do the things that he wanted to do. We did discuss that decision usually with great difficulty because what was at stake was so enormous. George's view was that if he had his right lung removed and the disease appeared in the left lung his death would actually be much more protracted, painful and difficult than if he ... had at least some function in the right lung ... in retrospect he was right ...

Other issues of conflict, was one time when he had quite a lot of pain in his right hip, he was worried about [it] ... He went to our GP who immediately sent him up to x-ray with a chitty to have an x-ray within hours of presenting . . . She was clearly, extremely worried about why he had a pain in his right hip. George himself had a very good instinct about his own state of health and he was convinced it was mechanical, that it was not a spread of the cancer . . . but he was compliant to a degree that he actually went up to the x-ray department, took the chitty, got on the couch and said to the radiologist, 'I hope this will only be one x-ray, I have had huge numbers of scans and x-rays, I have overdosed on radiation, I don't need anymore'. And she said, 'no I'm sorry George in order to get the information that we need, we have to take 6 or 7 x-rays of your leg'. At which point, he sat up . . . got off the couch and said, 'I'm not going to go through with this'. We then had a day of the GP chasing him around, really worried because x-ray had phoned her . . . And George won, George would not go for the x-ray instead he went down to our complementary health clinic and saw an osteopath who believed George's view that the pain in his hip was due to the fact that his diseased leg, the one which now contained the prosthesis was shorter than the healthy leg and was putting . . . a strain on the right hip, and he dealt with it that way. But that was a period of open defiance really he chose to go along the complementary route . . . He had a strong belief that he needed to address his own inner health and well being. And while the medical doctors could deal with his tumour, with chemo . . . what really George believed was that the real issue was his own inner . . . emotional health. And he felt that he had to work on that and he worked on that as a project throughout his illness. And it gave him great cause for hope – as well as despair and it gave him activity with strategies and things that he felt in control of.

I do feel that the model at the Royal Orthopaedic Hospital is also worth mentioning. The protocol was to be admitted to the Royal Orthopaedic, I think on the Sunday night, for biopsy probably on the Monday with the results of the biopsy being given in the middle of the week. We knew that George was very likely to be told whether or not he had cancer . . . what the extent of the spread might be, what the treatment protocols were going to be, and probably prognosis as well on the Wednesday. And . . . on the Wednesday . . . myself and George's dad, his brother and his girlfriend, were all in the hospital waiting so that we were all together and could hear the same news at the same time so that people weren't passing on reinterpreted messages. The consultants were extraordinarily busy because they were surgeons as well as oncologists and it wasn't until 9 o'clock at night that finally one of the three consultants had the time to come and talk to George. And the way he did it was to ask George first of all whether he wanted us all to be present or whether he wanted to be spoken to on his own. And George's choice was that he wanted to meet with the consultant on his own and to hear his

*news on his own for the first time and this took about 20 minutes.
So George was given enough time to ask questions and to ask for
clarifications. Then the consultant asked George's permission to go
over the same ground with the rest of us . . . And so at this point the
five of us . . . were in George's room with the consultant and he went
over exactly the same ground . . . as he'd already gone over with George
on his own, so we could all hear the same information given in the
same words at the same time. Now given that this was after a busy
day in the operating theatre, it was probably towards 10 at night by
the time this consultation had finished I am really full of admiration
for the way that was done and so important. Because for George, who
had had no experience of medical intervention at all up to that point,
apart from possibly the odd earache, it set a pattern that George then
followed for the rest of the illness, he always allowed us to hear the
information from the consultant direct but sometimes he wanted to
hear it first.*

The above account of George's diagnosis and treatment and his parents'
involvement suggests that the situation was managed with skill in the sharing of information. But as we saw in Chapter 1, the involvement of parents
in medical consultations may become more problematic when a son or
daughter reaches young adulthood. Young people in this age group are
legally entitled to be the recipient of medical information and may decide
not to share this with their parents. However, even earlier than this the
sharing of medical information and involvement in medical consultations
goes through a period of renegotiation. We have seen that during such
a period mothers in particular can feel excluded, for example when asked
to stay in the waiting room. They are however, unwilling to relinquish
involvement totally and will still expect a full account of the consultation.
Whether or not they get one may be a different matter, but having had the
responsibility for their child's health throughout their life until that point,
not to be involved would appear to result in some difficulty for the parents'
(mothers') ability to 'let go'.

Even when health-related decisions and medical consultations are routine
and pertain only to minor illness, parents can feel excluded if they are not
present at the GP's surgery or hospital appointment. However, if the young
person is away at university, such appointments may take place far from
home and parental involvement becomes less likely. Such a stage may
represent a sense of the young adults taking responsibility for their own
health. However, whilst the need for independence amongst young adults is
understandable, when the diagnosis is cancer related – or may be – such
exclusion can be particularly difficult for parents to manage and will
almost certainly result in their re-involvement with health-related decisions
– or at least an attempt at re-involvement.

When parents' concern is seen as interference

Parents can often be the first to spot the signs of ill health in their children – they have after all been doing just this all their children's lives. Yet when a son or daughter has reached young adulthood, it may not be deemed appropriate to suggest that medical advice is needed, or if it is suggested it can be ignored; if this is the case there appears to be very little a worried parent can do. We can see in the following extract from Helen V's narrative that her concern pre-dated by some time Simon's attempt to seek medical advice:

> I'd been nagging Simon for months about going to the Uni. medical service. One day when he was feeling really bad during a physics practice, he did go. I will never forget the Thursday afternoon when he came home from the physiotherapist's. His head hung down, he couldn't look at me, he just slumped. I'd been feeling concerned for months but had hesitated to interfere. He was 19, he was familiar with the medical system, and above all I was afraid that, if I suggested some course of action, he would reject it, teenage-style. Though Simon was very easygoing, he became understandably annoyed when I pestered him about his health. I remember once lifting up his T-shirt to see if he was wearing a singlet in the depths of winter – I'm not a subtle person. Simon was not impressed.
>
> (Helen V)

Concern over health issues may be a matter of some importance. But as we see here, parental concern can be a source of irritation to a young adult, even when directed towards what may become a matter of life and death. While his mother's anxiety was well-founded, suggestions from her to seek medical help were not welcomed. Simon's mother acknowledges how difficult it was to try not to be an 'interfering parent'.

> I was beside myself with concern for months, but did nothing effective because of this stupid notion that it would be better for him to 'own' the problem, to handle it his way. I felt he was too old to want me to accompany him to the doctor . . . All the . . . problems were made worse because I didn't know how to talk to Simon about personal things, and neither did Patrick.
>
> (Helen V)

Yet Helen V also says that she was aware that he was too young to know that he was not receiving good medical care. Again it seems that it is this precise life stage that creates a conflict in the need to be able to offer parental advice based on experience and better knowledge of medical services, and an inability to do so because of a fear it would be seen as 'interfering'. Again this relates directly to issues of independence discussed in Chapter 2.

Are they adults or children?

Sue documents the difficulty the parents in her self-help group had in accepting that their sick child was legally an adult.

> One mother in our group was horrified to hear a doctor telling her 23 year old daughter to her face that she would probably need a leg amputation. 'How could he say this to a child?' was her instinctive reaction. We found ourselves caught in a trap: emotionally, we of course all think of our offspring as our 'children', no matter what age. Legally, the situation is different.
>
> (Sue)

Having been the recipient of medical information for so many years there are bound to be problems when a parent hears a doctor impart such devastating news without the inclusion, permission or mediation of the parent. Sue continues her observations by pointing out that whilst being excluded from decision making, parents are still the ones to pick up the pieces and cope with the aftermath of those decisions.

> Unlike the parents of younger children, who were faced with making decisions on behalf of their underage children, we were often confronted with being isolated (hospitals, out-patient care, sometimes patients themselves) from the decision-making process, although we were all ultimately responsible for the day-to-day caring, nursing and financial support . . . Friends and family also tended to oscillate between viewing the young patients as child or adult, so that we lived in a continual state of not really knowing where we stood.
>
> (Sue)

Not only did the parents, friends and family not know if the young adults were 'adults' or 'children', it appears that some medical professionals were equally confused. Thus these young people who were neither child nor adult could quite arbitrarily find themselves in an inappropriate environment. Again using examples from the self-help group of parents, Sue observes:

> The 14 year old was a patient in an adult hospital, a 16 year old ended up in a children's hospital, two other older teenagers were the only 'young' patients on an adult oncology ward.
>
> (Sue)

Such problems would it seems make the process of hospital treatment even more difficult to endure. Whilst Sue reflects on the difficulties associated with a young adult being on a ward with much older patients, Denise suggests that being on a ward with children is equally problematic:

Laura was treated at the Royal Victoria Infirmary Newcastle by an excellent team of doctors and nurses on the Cancer Ward for Children. This was not our ideal ward – a teenager did not want to sleep next to a toddler in a ward filled with Teletubbies!!! Laura wanted privacy and different things during her stay in hospital. The staff did their best under very difficult circumstances and fortunately Laura had relatively short stays compared to some children. . . . She made it very clear that she needed to be in control and make decisions. We like many parents found this difficult but always respected her wishes no matter how much we were hurting inside – Laura was a remarkable, intelligent young lady and we owed it to her . . . In October '97 they opened a Teenage Cancer Unit at Newcastle which made such a difference to the patients and their families. The staff and facilities were just unbelievable and we really did have help and support from so many different sources including other parents should you want it.

(Denise)

Denise, like other parents, found this relinquishing of control difficult. Laura was only 15 when first diagnosed, and the dichotomy between the children's ward and the 'adult' decisions must have only served to further confuse matters. However, when Laura was placed on a more appropriate ward with other young adults, we can see that this made a considerable difference to her parents, and we assume to her as well.

The difficulties experienced by Lynn's son, Simon R, in intensive care are related here:

They [intensive care nurses] normally look after an unconscious patient and are not used to dealing with alive and moving patients fighting for their lives. Their . . . routine was being interfered with by this bloody cheeky patient who refused to lie still and be quiet and demanded attention.

(Lynn)

This quotation suggests that the staff were unused to caring for young people whose needs are different from those usually cared for on an ITU ward, again reinforcing the need for a specialist understanding of young adults.

Despite the fact that Joyce's daughter, Jill was 22 when she was diagnosed with osteosarcoma, and 24 when she died, it is clear that her parents protected her from full knowledge of the seriousness of her condition:

We never mentioned death, we role played for one another. The nearest she came to saying anything was one day, she said 'I am very ill mum'. I said 'I know darling'. She liked to hold our hands. She said she took our strength and it made her feel better. It was the worst time in our lives, seeing our daughter slowly dying and not being able to stop it

from happening . . . I gave up my full-time job, when Jill was diagnosed with cancer. I worked part-time and made it fit in with our
journeys to Manchester. The last month I took indefinite leave, to
nurse her at home. I found her pain level and kept her pain free with
morphine. She was still alert, not frightened and happy to be at home.

(Joyce)

A number of the young adults in these narratives have died at home, and
as in the extract from Joyce's narrative, we see that this is something that
was valued by her son or daughter. Although 'place of death' is an important issue for both parents and young adult, it is mentioned only in passing
in many of the narrative contributions. However, where it is mentioned it
appears that it has been the specific wish of young adults to die at home,
and that at some expense – both emotional and financial – parents accommodate this wherever possible. This may in part be due to the limited
number of specialist facilities that care for young adults in hospitals. Whilst
there are some Teenage Cancer Wards there are not enough for all young
people who need them, and their geographical proximity to some patients
may be problematic. Some of the confusions over how the medical knowledge is shared may well be overcome in units where there are experts in
caring for this age group.

Added to the confusion and ambiguity already documented are the
problems associated with the 'blame' that may be laid on parents over
treatment decisions. We have already seen that parents can be, and often
are, excluded from decision making, yet this does not stop their son or
daughter from blaming them for the consequences.

Alex also insisted that he had never wanted to undergo treatment in
the first place, but that we parents had coerced him into it (although he
alone was responsible for signing the forms of consent, which he did
without protest), and he just wanted to be left to die in peace. As a
result, he was aggressive towards us parents and sometimes to his
bewildered brother and sister as well . . .

(Sue)

Who owns the medical information?

Further confusion and distress can be caused by medical professionals'
adherence to patient confidentiality, which may or may not be understood
by the family. Indeed from the following quotation, it seems that it may not
even be understood by the medical professionals themselves:

Because Alex was of age, the doctors were not allowed to divulge any
information about his situation to us unless they had his permission in
writing. Sadly, they did not tell us this, so it took us a while to work

out what was happening. Further confusion was caused as individual staff sometimes broke the rule. Things only improved when Alex finally decided that we parents might be put in the picture, as he grudgingly admitted that we were 'somehow practically involved'!

(Sue)

Charlotte's account of Sean being informed of his terminal diagnosis seems to indicate that she was asked to be there specifically to hear this news:

> When Sean and I were told it was definitely terminal by the doctor, he said he had thought about death. We were told very nicely with a nurse present. There was a lot of eye contact inter-changing between us all. He was disappointed and we both cried afterwards – not a lot. Sean said 'oh well, there is no point in getting upset'. I put my arms around him and hugged him and said 'I had wanted to do that for ages'. The oncologist had wanted me present when speaking to Sean, so I knew what he was going to say. Doctors do not see relatives for trivial reasons.
>
> (Charlotte)

This encounter appears to have led to a closeness between Charlotte and Sean that allowed her to express her feelings. Perhaps she was afraid that if she had taken such a demonstrative stance earlier, Sean would have interpreted it as confirmation of a bleak prognosis. Yet, to some extent this doctor's procedures contradict the indications we have had that if the young adult is 'of age' they will be given the medical information directly and choose whether they share it with their parents.

Sue B faced a similar situation. In the following account of her son Paul being given news of whether his cancer had spread, we see that she was asked by the nurses if she wished to be present, but it was Paul who decided that he wanted to be on his own:

> Two nurses asked me if I wanted to join him but Paul wanted to face it on his own. I suppose I would have said silly things but I wished at the time I had been with him. I know now that once again his courage was far greater than anything I could ever come near.
>
> (Sue B)

It is evident in the extract that Sue B found being excluded difficult, and much like Helen V, who felt that her son would be better with his friends, we see that Paul's mother belittles her contribution by suggesting that she would have said 'silly things'. Perhaps what she means here is that she would have done as many mothers in these circumstances would have done and become upset, asking a myriad of questions and possibly causing her son embarrassment.

The way in which Denise C was informed of her son's diagnosis also reflects a lack of certainty as to the ownership of information:

> Things got off to a bad start when the diagnosis of Alexander's cancer was delivered to me alone, over the telephone by a consultant who should have known better than to impart such devastating news in this way and bearing in mind that Alexander was 19 years old also breached confidentiality.
>
> (Denise C)

The insensitivity demonstrated in this example is a manifestation not only of bad practice in relation to Alexander's age and legal status as an adult, but reflects an unacceptable approach to imparting bad news no matter what age the patient is. Whether Alexander's age was a contributing factor here we do not know, but it may be that with less confusion over the ownership of information the situation might have been handled differently.

However, there appear to be occasions when the situation is even more uncertain and negotiable. Despite her son being of age, Brenda went to considerable pains to prevent him being informed of the seriousness of his condition, fearing that if he were told he would give up and refuse treatment:

> Although reeling from the shock of being told he was terminally ill, I was adamant that I did not want my son to know he was dying. As he was technically an adult this was a constant battle in the early stages to persuade his consultant, hospital medical team, hospice staff, district nurse, etc. that I was right to take this course. I however, was convinced that it was the only way to get him through it. Had he not been confident of a cure he could never have got through the dreadful weeks of chemotherapy, radiotherapy, and isolation treatment he had to endure. He hated it when a counsellor showed him too much compassion in the hospital. He said she was 'like the kiss of death' and refused to see her again. We persuaded him to be admitted to a local hospice for a couple of days since he was still in unbearable pain which made him yell uncontrollably at times. I was finding his anguish and agony so very difficult to watch and the hospice was sure that with the correct drugs they could alleviate some of the pain. However, the elderly dying patients around him had a very depressing effect on him. He never thought he would die in these early days and I knew that once he lost his will to fight on we would never be able to deal with his increasing moods and depression. I did win my case in the end but was always worried that some well-meaning medic would tell him that his was a hopeless case.
>
> (Brenda)

We see two things happening here. The first is that Brenda has managed, despite Miles being of age, to persuade the medical professionals not to divulge his prognosis to him – thus flying in the face of current orthodoxies about the 'open awareness context'. She refers to this as a 'constant battle', and she must have been in a continual state of concern that a well-meaning member of staff would let slip how seriously ill he actually was. To keep such information secret must have added considerably to the stress Brenda was under. In addition Brenda refers to the fact that Miles was on an inappropriate ward, surrounded by elderly, dying patients who brought down his morale. Again we see that life stage here directly affected Miles's ability to respond positively to the medical environment, a point also made by Denise, Sue and other parents in her self-help group.

Moira also made a decision not to tell her son of the very bleak prognosis when Alasdair, who had osteosarcoma, was diagnosed with terminal secondaries:

> We decided after much discussion with GPs the nurses and Marie Curie nurses who helped us look after him and Heather (Macmillan nurse) not to tell him he was dying, unless he asked. He was still so hopeful for the future, getting back to college with a carer and so on, we couldn't 'shoot him down' as it were. We will always be grateful to the army of nurses who made it possible to keep Alasdair at home until he was taken to St. Andrews Hospice in Airdrie for pain control. It was only to be for a few days, but it proved impossible to get it controlled. The doctor said a lot of it was mental agony. I had tried to get Alasdair to talk about how he felt, tried to get him to tell me what he was thinking, tried to drop gently hints about the way things were going, but he wouldn't 'bite'. I encouraged him to talk to the wonderful hospice staff, but he wouldn't or couldn't?
>
> (Moira)

Despite the fact that a decision not to tell Alasdair about the seriousness of his condition had been taken, it does seem that at some level his mother wanted to share this information with him before he died and we see her attempts to get him to 'bite'. It is perhaps a similar situation that we see in the following extract where Claire indicates that it was her daughter Laura W who did not want the burden of the prognosis, but neither did she want her parents to have that knowledge:

> During what was to be her final fortnight, she told us not to ask for a prognosis, as she didn't want to know, and knew that she would pick up the cues from us. We knew that she was receiving palliative care (but not that death was only days away). My first reaction to her 'order' was that I was pleased that she had not picked up what we knew, by my demeanour. This was swiftly followed by feeling that

I had betrayed her, and then by a resolution not to give away anything. And I continue to wrestle with that – all those expressions of love and gratitude I wanted to share with her, but held back, knowing that even at this stage, her antennae were finely tuned and would have interpreted any such expressions as farewells. I was even more reticent than usual, in case she picked up my signals. Part of my response was probably that I was protecting myself – when here she was, a 21 year old and dying – protecting myself.

(Claire)

Here it is apparent that Claire's knowledge of the bleakness of the prognosis was something of a burden and having successfully concealed her reactions from her daughter, she felt as though she had 'betrayed' her.

However, the balance of the ownership of the information appeared to change during the course of Michael T's illness. Whilst Michael T appeared to be in receipt of the medical information from the time of his diagnosis when he was 16 – perhaps because there was a hopeful outlook – at the age of 18 when he was diagnosed with terminal cancer, the consultant told his mother not to pass on the information:

It is very hard when you are on your own to make your mind up what is right for your child. But because Michael turned 16 years old in January, 1996, he made his own mind up about what to do. Then in April 1998 we had to go back to Leeds to see [the consultant] and did more scans. And he told us that they had found another lump on Michael's lungs and they couldn't do anymore chemotherapy because they gave Michael the strongest one before. [The doctor] asked Michael if he could have a word with me in private. Then [he] told me that Michael only had months to live. That broke my heart because [he] told me not to tell Michael.

(Elizabeth)

Elizabeth was a single parent. Whilst being married or having a partner in such circumstances might in itself cause discord at times (see Chapter 8), being alone with the burden of such knowledge brings its own difficulties. Elizabeth herself acknowledges that when you are on your own it is very hard to decide what is the right thing to do. Having a partner may in fact not make the decision easier, particularly if there is disagreement about the best way to manage the situation. So perhaps what Elizabeth is also feeling here is a sense of aloneness, carrying the whole burden of her son's terminal cancer diagnosis without a co-parent to share it with.

However, when a month later Michael T's condition had worsened and he was being cared for at home with the support of his GP and social worker, his mother recounts the following:

Michael was talking to . . . the social worker and he said he'd got four wishes:

1 To be at home.
2 He wanted his mum and brother to be there.
3 To die in his sleep like his grandad did.
4 And to be buried with his grandad.

He got all four wishes; they all came true for him . . . Michael told his brother two days before he passed away that he loved his brother and goodbye. He even asked a friend who he only knew for four months, would he and John, Michael's brother, carry his coffin because he never wanted to go on the trolley.

(Elizabeth)

It seems as if Michael T needed to know that he was dying so that he could make clear his wishes. How could he have articulated these wishes if he had not known that he would die?

Michael T was 18 when he died, but Christine, also a single parent decided that her son Tony, although only 15, should be informed of his condition. However, Christine also attempted to reassure Tony that it was a condition he would survive:

I didn't really know what to do, because I thought shall I tell Tony or not? But 'cause I'm on my own with him he knew there was something wrong . . . I think 'cause he knew I was upset and because he said to me 'why are you crying?' 'Cause you know, 'cause he obviously knew oh gosh something's wrong. And, I did tell him, but I put it like 'well you've got cancer but it's just like having meningitis you know, you are gonna be OK, I'll be here for you and everything . . .' And all the treatment he's had, going through the hospital, going through Christie's, it's always been both of us, we've both been there.

(Christine)

Tony is now of age, but he and his mother still share the information on his illness, and he has as yet shown no desire to keep it from her. Alex too made it clear that he wanted to be told the truth about his condition, no matter how bleak the prognosis:

Alex wanted to be told the truth. No matter how unpalatable it was. It was imperative that he had the facts so he could continue to make decisions and remain in control, which in turn meant dying with dignity and respect. We had always spoken openly about the possibility of his death, and now that it was a certainty, we saw no reason for changing tactics. The doctors in Birmingham told him the score, honestly and directly, and then sent in a team of supporters to help with the repercussions. Doctors at our hospital in Germany avoided the issue and offered no back-up services. For us, the first approach was the better one.

I had to be very insistent before the (German) doctor was prepared to answer my question about what exactly would be the cause of death in the end (asphyxiation) and what could be done to alleviate it (sedation). But this information was vital to Alex – he was no longer afraid of death, but he was afraid of dying. He was tremendously relieved to hear that he would not have to choke to death while fully conscious.

We had many chats about life, death and how we would manage afterwards without him. For us, this was the right way. Alex was calm and unworried, and knew that we were ready to let him go, which made his death much easier for him.

(Sue)

Here we see Sue contrasting experiences of the difference in approach between Germany and England where Alex was treated. Clearly she and Alex preferred the honest and open approach they experienced in England; indeed such honesty helped to allay his fears about what death might entail. He was also reassured that his family would be all right after his death, and Sue believes that this helped him in a calmer and easier death than had these issues remained unaddressed. We see also that his siblings were kept informed, though Sue does reflect on the fact that whilst they appeared at 18 and 21 to be 'grown up', they too were at the 'between stage' so relevant to all aspects of this book.

Young people who are diagnosed while away at university may have to cope with the diagnosis on their own, and this can be problematic for both the young adult and the parents, as we see from Jeremy and Lesley's account of their son Timothy's diagnosis of testicular cancer:

From September to December he had been having chest problems and was treated by the University Medical Centre for pleurisy. No medical tests were done to confirm this diagnosis, it was only when Timothy finally collapsed at 02.00 hours coming home from a party that he was taken to casualty at the Royal Berkshire Hospital for a check up. It was at this point that chest x-rays were finally taken and Timothy was advised that his condition was serious and merited further tests. He was told he had cancer, by the doctor, when he had no family around him to discuss the problem and wandered around the streets of Reading before going back to the hospital to be admitted for yet more tests . . . His flat mates were very careful as to what they said over the telephone, and the hospital would only confirm which ward he was on. The sister said he was down for further tests and would ring when he was back on the ward. Timothy had left instructions that he would break the news, and he would decide what we were to know, a policy he followed throughout his illness . . . He was initially given a 20%

survival rate by Christie's, Timothy later admitted that the survival rate had doubled since leaving Reading!! This is when he advised us that the doctors were under orders to tell him everything first and he would decide what we were to be told. It was very hard to watch our child take all this on himself. We wanted to wrap him up in cotton wool, but he needed space to fight it in his own way.

(Jeremy and Lesley)

Here we have a combination of factors to be dealt with by the parents, on the one hand the fact that their son was diagnosed so far from home, and on the other that he made it explicit that he would decide what his parents were told about his condition. Again this relates strongly to the discussion in Chapter 2 on independence. Jeremy and Lesley recognize their need to protect Timothy, but have to respect his 'need for space'. George too was diagnosed whilst at university, but it seems that he was well supported by the doctor at the university Medical Centre. He was still, however, waiting for his parents' arrival and demonstrably glad to see them.

One account where the confusions and complexities appear to have been resolved is given by Denise C:

During Alexander's illness, we always tried to be guided by him, and respect his wishes as to decision-making and steps to take. It was very difficult as he was over 18 and 'legally not bound to our apron strings'. How to keep in the background and yet want to shower him with our parental protection? How would the doctors feel about him taking control? How did they feel about us being there? After he died, the chief consultant did compliment us on getting the balance right without intruding. That was good to hear – At the time, one acts in good faith but never quite sure whether it's the right thing to do. We needn't have worried – Alexander led the way and was congratulated by the medics for his forthrightness and clinic management.

(Denise C)

Whilst Denise C raises many of the same issues and questions as other parents, it seems that in retrospect she can look back on the management of the situation and know that with sensitivity to her son's needs an appropriate balance between independence and privacy was achieved.

Reflections

Many of the issues raised through these narratives relate to the confusing and problematic nature of the sharing of medical information. This however, did not appear to be a problem between George and his parents.

George's mother tells us that despite the fact that he wanted to be given the information directly and on his own, he also wanted his parents to be in full receipt of the same information. This would sometimes necessitate the doctor relating it twice, once to George on his own and once more together. However, this did not appear to be problematic. What does seem to have been more of an issue in George's story, which has not been raised to any great extent in the narratives, is a disagreement about treatment regimes. George's mother acknowledges that there were occasions when she wanted to proceed with aggressive treatment and he did not. She wanted him to be put on the drug trial and also to have surgery to remove his lung. On both occasions he resisted, as was his right, but it left his mother in a state of helpless anxiety. He took a similar stand against having the six or seven x-rays on his hip and refused, preferring to trust his instincts and seek advice from a complementary therapist. Whilst she acknowledges that ultimately his decision was probably the best one for him and that he knew best how his illness should be managed, at the time the situation was exceedingly difficult for his mother to manage.

Again life stage is crucial, when parents have until relatively recently been used to making medical decisions on behalf of their son or daughter, usually in relation to minor illnesses, to relinquish this control over cancer can be traumatic. Brannen, Dodd, Oakley and Storey (1994) document the trouble that mothers in particular, have in letting go of the ownership of their children's health and health-related decisions. So once again we can see the exacerbation of the problem in relation to life stage and the struggle for control and ownership of medical information and decisions that are a part of the understandable bid for independence and the young person's legal right.

Health professionals are also heavily involved in the issues discussed in this chapter. Whilst in some cases, such as George's, they appear to have handled the situation with sensitivity, giving George the information first and then sharing it with his parents with his consent, this clarity and sensitivity does not seem to have been the case in many of the examples from the narratives. The legal situation is clear, but it is also clear that it is on occasion negotiated between parents and medical staff. It is difficult to make any recommendations about the 'best' way to handle the situation, but we have seen examples of confusion, which need to be clarified. Perhaps, where appropriate, a frank discussion between all parties at an early stage establishing ground rules for communication is needed. On the other hand it may be necessary to 'play it by ear' making judgements as the illness and its treatment develop. Thornes (2001: 55) argues that the family of a young person should be included in the care plan (with permission) to a greater extent than is usual in adult services as even after the age of majority many young people will be tightly linked to the family both in practical and emotional terms. However, the key must be good communication – between medical staff and the young adult, between young adults and their parents and between the parents and the health professionals.

Much work has been carried out on the importance of 'awareness' in relation to dying patients. Glaser and Strauss (1965) who analysed the social actions engaged in by health professionals found various 'awareness contexts': 'closed' where the doctor and patient conspire to keep the truth from the family; 'suspicion' where the patient tries to extract the truth; 'mutual pretence' where both sides know the patient is dying but no one mentions it; and 'open' where there is open communication between the patient, the family and the health professionals (Glaser and Strauss 1965, cited in Walter 1994: 31). As Walter says, since this study there has been a major movement away from the belief that keeping patients in ignorance is desirable to the belief that an 'open' model assists patients in making decisions about their remaining life.

The following studies charted by Clark and Seymour (1999) show that whilst significant advances in the field have been made, there are still areas of concern in relation to practice. Field (1989), whilst demonstrating that practices have changed in relation to the disclosure of terminal illness since the early work of Glaser and Strauss (1965), suggests that nursing in some settings still encourages pretence. Robbins's (1998) comparison of the work of Perakyla (1989) and Hunt (1991), both of whom identified a range of roles adopted by staff when dealing with dying patients, observes that such roles may be used as strategies to manage the stress associated with the care of dying people.

However, even if there is an explicit adoption of an 'open awareness' policy, the breaking of bad news is a complex matter. According to De Valck, Bensing and Bruynooghe (2001) it remains unclear how the disclosure of such news is related to the health professionals' attitudes. Three main models are identified by Donovan (1993) as non-disclosure, full-disclosure and individualized disclosure. The first assumes a paternalistic stance based on the avoidance of evoking fear and anxiety in the patient, the second stresses the ethical right of each individual to know the truth and the last recognizes that the amount of information should be tailored to the 'preferences' of each patient.

Results of research amongst medical students undertaken by De Valck and colleagues (2001) suggest that approaches to breaking bad news are related to different global attitudes, and that there is a gender divide, with women being more likely than men to adopt a collaborative model in the patient–physician relationship – a finding supported by Hall and Roter (1998). But even the full-disclosure model can be approached in different ways; for example, full-disclosure may be approached in either a bio-medical/detached manner or with a much more person-centred psychosocially-oriented attitude.

So it appears that whilst there is much debate in this area and an apparently increasing acceptance of the importance of 'awareness', practice will vary according to the social setting and individual practitioner's model and world view. When coupled with the issues of ambiguity raised in this chapter by the transition from childhood to adulthood we cannot be surprised at the range of experiences expressed.

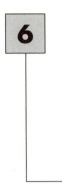

6 The effect on siblings: managing conflicting demands

George's story

We were acutely aware that there were three sons not just one who had had their lives thrown into turmoil by the cancer diagnosis and were very conscious that they needed to survive George's illness. And I think from the start, I was aware that George might not survive, but that Jonathan and David must survive his illness. And that it was very important that their lives were not thrown off course because they were both at fairly crucial stages, as young people are in their education. David was 11 at the time of diagnosis in the top class at junior school, about to make the transition from primary to secondary schooling, which he actually did. He began grammar school while George was recovering at home from the surgery for his leg. And his first term at grammar school was against the backdrop of George having the remaining four sessions of chemotherapy, being in hospital for three or four days and then home for about three weeks being extremely sick, sometimes in his bedroom for 10 days without even being able to come downstairs. David appears to have coped extremely well with George's illness and I think one big reason for this is George's own awareness of David's vulnerability . . . However poorly George felt, however bad a day he had had, he would always make an enormous effort for David after school to be interested in what he'd done, to watch TV programmes if that's all he had the energy to do . . . even when George was within weeks of dying and it was David's 15th birthday. George was up and dressed and downstairs helping David assemble his hi fi equipment that he'd been given for his birthday, before David went to school. Now George didn't normally get up till lunch-time. He was acutely aware of how important it was for him to be unselfish I suppose where David was concerned and he was absolutely brilliant. Also, he needed David because David was the one person who didn't treat him with kid gloves, who was naturally relaxed with him as were David's two special friends Joe and George. They could come in and they could joke and they could lark around and they could be silly with George, they could be rude to him, they could tease him in a way that nobody else could. So having a younger sibling around, from George's point of view was a real bonus. David doesn't ever talk about his feelings during George's illness. I think he took his cue from George which was that, 'I'm going to beat this illness and I am going to get better' and I think David believed that throughout the illness. So he wasn't subject to the acute anxiety and stomach-churning anguish that Geoff and I experienced throughout most of the four years. When we went to Birmingham we were low key. David didn't know what was at stake and we wanted him to be kept from that . . . we were very lucky in that we lived in a very settled community where we have been for 25 years where there are families and friends around who moved in, in a way that, I think David didn't even notice really . . . one particular friend from London came to stay as often as she could, Geoff's sister came as often as she could, and one of George's friends, Amy, would take over housekeeping in our absence. So quite often if we weren't in the house, David's routine carried on with other people staying and we've always been a fairly sort of open house anyway and his dad goes away for work quite often. So it wasn't unusual to have people staying . . . it was unusual to have me away, his mum, but not unusual to have his dad away. And I think because he was so well supported, David survived it extremely well.

What I saw as important was to make sure that David was all right here . . . and the fact that his two special friends lived very, very close by and their families are family friends meant that he had two families where he could always retreat to when the going was tough at home. We always said we were extremely fortunate in that these families did not protect their youngsters who were David's age from George's illness. They were allowed to come and go and they were allowed to see George, however poorly he was, in a way perhaps some families would have not wanted to happen. So David's life changed as little as possible . . . He hardly ever came down to Birmingham because . . . times in Birmingham were tense and very difficult and George was usually quite poorly. I don't think George particularly wanted to see him, I think he came maybe once or twice. But it all ran so smoothly, I can't even remember the details of it, the whole support network of family and friends just swung into place and there seemed to be a seamless sort of movement really between Birmingham and Lancaster. And I don't think David noticed that we weren't here and to have . . . the task of protecting him was good for

all of us because it meant that we tried to be up-beat at least in a
public way.

Jonathan was, I think, affected a lot more. He was older and at the
time of George's diagnosis was in Florence at the European University
Institute doing a Masters in European Law. He had taken a villa in the
Tuscan hills for the summer of '95 in order to write up his dissertation
before coming back to England and starting Bar School. When we got
George's diagnosis within hours we made contact with Jonathan, or at
least Jonathan's housemates, Jonathan was in Venice for the weekend, to
let him know what was happening. And he immediately came home. And
he was with us in Birmingham within 48 hours of George's admission to
Birmingham and he was there for the diagnosis. He stayed around for 2
or 3 weeks until George began the chemo. He went back to Florence to
try to pick up where he left off, but I don't think he stayed more than a
week or 10 days, he just couldn't. So he came back to Lancaster with
his dissertation unwritten intending to write it over the summer while
George had chemo and surgery and before he started Law School,
in fact he couldn't settle at all, he just didn't manage to do any work
or very little work. But he just managed . . . to submit in February of
the following year while he was still at Bar School. But it really was a
miracle that he got his Masters at all. However, he did go to Bar School
and he did get through Bar School, and I don't know how he managed it.
He also got a pupillage at a prestigious chambers. But yet my memory
of it, whenever anything of major significance has happened to George
whether it was a particularly difficult check-up or a particular piece of
treatment or holiday or special occasion or anything of that nature,
Jonathan was always either here or in Birmingham, wherever he needed
to be. And looking back now, I don't know how he did it. He also got
married and I just look at Jonathan with amazement really as to how he
kept his life going, how he has managed to build up a successful career
as a barrister and to have managed to settle into a happy and fulfilling
married relationship under such difficult circumstances. After George
died, Jonathan was the most outwardly affected of all of us, he really
struggled, he was immensely angry at the injustice of what had happened
and it was having an effect on his life in all sorts of areas. But he was
very fortunate in that our hospice social worker put him in touch with
a counsellor through one of the London hospices who turned out to be
absolutely excellent. And the timing was right and the personality was
right and a period of maybe 8 or so counselling sessions seemed to be
enormously beneficial to Jonathan. He also went to counselling during
part of George's illness . . . with Bacup, one of the cancer charities in
London. So he did have opportunities to speak to people outside of the
family, and he was very well supported by friends. Two particular close
friends from when he was very young had both lost parents to cancer and

really knew what Jonathan was facing in a very personal way and were extremely supportive and he was able I think to share it with them. And he also had the support of his new partner and now wife, Helen, who I think took a huge burden. This was a family that she'd come into in a period of crisis, she hadn't known us before George was ill. She met Jonathan, as George was beginning his first lot of treatment and it's sad for me that she didn't know us when life was different before our family became disrupted and I suppose fragmented by George's illness. But it seems to me very important that Jonathan has a wife who knows what he went through during the four years of George's illness and treatment. Because somebody who met him after that period I think wouldn't understand what a massive event it is in his life and will always be in his life. I'm not too sure what the longer term holds for David who is now 17, because David is going to make a lot of relationships with people who will have no experience of George and will not know what his life was like from the age of 11 to 16. And I'm not even sure how much he will be able to articulate about that time. I trust he will find that he can talk about it if he needs to. But I don't think the bereavement journey is yet over for David because I think he still has to, in a sense, go back over in his own mind those years between 11 and 16 from a mature perspective when he was protected a lot from what was going on. As an adult he will look back and know that there were things around of which he wasn't aware . . .

George's mother acknowledges that her family was in a relatively fortunate position, with strong family relationships, material advantages and well supported within the community. This, however, is not always the case. At the point of diagnosis or during the course of the illness, families may also experience other traumatic life events, such as bereavement, divorce, illness or moving house. Events such as these, recounted by some respondents, clearly make the management of the cancer journey even more stressful to all members of the family, have an additional impact on the siblings and in turn place an even heavier burden on the parents.

The siblings of young adults are also likely to be in a similar age range, in need of parental guidance and attention (whether they admit it or not) and profoundly affected by the illness of their brother or sister. We saw in Chapter 1 that siblings manifest many feeling and emotions, some of which may be well founded, such as fear for their brother or sister's life, or feeling marginalized or excluded from their parents' concern. However, they may also feel unfounded guilt or resentment that has to be managed. But how do the parents cope with the balancing act that has to be implemented in caring for a seriously ill child, whilst also remembering the needs of their other children? It appears from the account given by George's mother that the family managed this balance well, but she admits that the social support network which swung into action to care for George's younger brother was invaluable. Had they been more socially isolated or had David not had such close friends able to care for him the situation might have been different. In the case of George's family, it was it seems his older brother, already away from home and studying abroad who had most difficulty in dealing with George's illness and death. Although Jonathan succeeded at Bar School his mother says that it was amazing that he got his Masters degree which was so seriously disrupted by George's illness.

Siblings and life-stage

Echoing George's story, Helen V points out that siblings may also be facing other demanding life-stage challenges, such as exams or professional training. Her older daughter, coincidentally also a law student, shares some of the experiences of George's older brother:

> Obviously it's tough on sibs of any age, but for one of ours it was terrible. Sarah hardly knew what was going on. It was almost easier with our older daughter. She has an intellectual disability and so we were forced to simplify. I just don't know what it's been like for her . . . Sarah was at a critical stage in her studies. Law students here are selected by firms before they begin their final year. So these were the exams that would decide her future, and she missed them by coming to London. She sat for supplementaries in January while still overwhelmed. Later, she told me that for six months after Simon's death, she'd lost all her motivation and could hardly study. In the end, she was taken on by a firm she liked, but it was just a terrible time for her to go through this experience. She still suffers, of course.
>
> (Helen V)

Sue makes a similar observation and draws on the experiences of the members of her self-help group to demonstrate that life-stage issues affect siblings as well as young adults with cancer:

> Illness at this time of life will almost certainly interfere with crucial exams, job hunting or training programmes, if not for the patients themselves then very probably for the siblings. This poses a higher stress level than in other age groups who are more likely to be established in a career or not yet facing decisive stages at school.
>
> (Sue)

Sue also points out that offers of help are more problematic (though no less welcome or necessary) in this age group:

> All of us felt very alone at some time or another – as of course other groups will do too. But we found that because we no longer had very

small children (or not even children at all, but 'adults'), people around us either did not perceive any particular need to offer practical help (which we all felt we could have done with) or did not know how to help. After all, it's easy to offer to take young siblings to the play-ground, but what do you do with older teenagers?

(Sue)

It seems from this extract that what Sue is saying is that all the confusion and ambivalence associated with the experiences of a young adult with cancer may also affect the siblings in the family and impact on the parents. This can result in a situation where the whole family can be thrown into, not only an emotional crisis, but also a practical crisis. Sue continues her reflections by considering how to tell Alex's siblings that he would die:

I did my best to prepare his siblings too, by telling them his death was imminent, making sure that they had plenty of opportunities to be with their brother individually, even if they didn't manage to say fare-well in so many words. I tried to involve them in all the stages, from learning that they were helping Alex by being with him and not aban-doning him, to buying him a computer game that might make him smile, to being with him at the moment of death as he wished, particip-ating in the funeral arrangements and having an equal say in how to plan the grave.

But it is the same problem. Just because they are legally adults, an eighteen-year old and a mentally-ill twenty-year old are still very young and continue to need considerable emotional support. So more dip-lomatic efforts are required! And again, there is little appreciation of their agony and pain: 'they are grown up then' is the reaction I get time after time.

(Sue)

Whilst Sue has clearly taken great care to involve Alex's siblings, and to help them participate in his illness and death it seems that their life stage, similar to that of their brother, also has an impact largely unappreciated by those outside the family. Here we also see a family coping with additional pressures, such as the mental illness of Alex's sister Natalie.

The anxiety generated in siblings

Having had a sibling die or experience life-threatening illness at such a young age may also result in acute anxiety amongst siblings who then fear for their own health as Sue's concern for her younger son, Benjamin, demonstrates:

Frightening for him until today is the thought that he might also get cancer. Every so often he is under the weather, often admits to 'bumps and lumps' of unidentified origin, and is worried. When this happens, I try to take his fear seriously and not tell him he's just imagining things, but at the same time make reassuring noises about how highly unlikely it would be before dispatching him to the doctor's for professional confirmation. I hope that with time, he will be less frightened.

(Sue)

What difficult balances to strike: on the one hand not appearing dismissive, whilst on the other reassuring. But since Alex's death Sue has had cause for concern over Benjamin's health. Two years after Alex died, Benjamin did become ill – the illness was not cancer nor indeed life-threatening – however, Sue's experience of supporting Benjamin through relatively minor surgery was profoundly affected by her previous experience with Alex. In the following extract she speaks of mental slippage between the past and the present, not being able to remember why she was at the hospital, or with which son. She was transported back to Alex's terminal illness and the suffering they both endured at the same hospital where Benjamin was being treated:

the surgeon might have finally – yesterday morning – succeeded in freeing Benjamin from the rocky pile-up and his gall bladder, but being thrown back into the hospital routine, mopping up sick bowls, holding a sticky hand under the sheets, watching the level in the urinal catheter slowly rise and being confronted with one of Alex's doctors who has switched workplaces makes my legs go weak and addles my brain and leaves me amazed that we ever got through a total of twelve months in hospital. I think – I hope – he can be discharged tomorrow as I really cannot stand much more of this although it is on the surface all quite harmless but I am memory weary and every little insignificant detail takes on magnified proportions . . . excellent decor right down to the psychologically uplifting yellow striped duvet cover which Alex had in his last week too . . . And Wolfgang is busy every afternoon this week being an Intel Master Teacher (Power Point!) and is glad because he cannot face coming in to visit his stitched up son any more than I can, but he has an alibi. Natty came for a while on Tuesday evening – before the surgeon/operateur had managed to get his hands on him – and asked me how I can bear it and she keeps thinking of Alex's leg with its 75 cm long wound. Laura comes a few hours after the op and is shocked at what she sees and doesn't understand about the tube in his stomach and can't cope alone and so I have to stay with her in the room until she goes. So the only person missing is Alex and I muddle up my sons and tell the nurse when I go that Alex is alone for a while and he gives me a funny look. So now I must drag myself back up there and keep Benjamin – yes Benjamin – company although I have but crumbs of comfort left for him as I have irretrievably used up a lifetime's supply for my firstborn.

(Sue)

Sue's account is more about how she coped with illness in her younger son rather than how Benjamin himself related to his brother's illness. But Iris documents the effect of Matthew's illness on his brother and sister:

His brother was so very close to Mat. He was away at university for three years, and said he always had Mat on his mind. There was always that fear as I have explained before. Nathan always believed in God. His belief took a U-turn, when Mat became ill. To this day he doubts that there is a God. He still believes that there is something more powerful than us, but cannot explain what is it. He says that he feels relieved that Mat is dead. There is no more pain for any of us. We know that Mat is better off. Nathan feels comfortable with life now. He misses Mat more than any of us. He has never been able to mourn. He doesn't cry anymore over anything. He has built this wall around himself, trying to be strong, but scared of the wall crumbling and himself with it. At 27 years old he admits he is frightened of crying, because he doesn't think he will be able to stop.

When Mat died Nathan was the one who remained strong. He took over, and did the things his dad should have done, because his dad has been unable to cope with losing Mat.

Mat's sister too has withdrawn into herself. She has become hurtful on occasions. She tried to be adult, but deep down there is still a little girl who hurts. Her life was thrown into turmoil when Mat first got sick at the age of twelve. She was nine years old and because I was at the hospital with Mat a lot, she spent over a year virtually living with her nan. She got spoiled and it shows. She had to sit her A-levels just two days after Mat died, and didn't do as well as she expected. She has, however, continued on to university where she is training to be a teacher – her lifetime ambition. She hates being too far from home and has obtained a place (doing her PGCE) at Bath, around 120 miles away. I am holding my breath until she finally gets there. I am afraid for her.

(Iris)

Whilst Iris presents this moving account of the effects on Matthew's brother and sister, we have to remember that she has had to cope with these effects on the family. While mourning the loss of her son, she speaks of Matthew's sister 'being hurtful'. There is no blame attached to this observation, and she attributes the effects on the fact that she had to be absent much of the time when Matthew was ill, and that his sister was 'spoiled' while in the care of her grandparents. Is she to some extent accepting 'blame' for his sister's behaviour, does she feel responsible because she had to leave her to be with Matthew? Iris's son has been equally but differently affected. Iris also says that her surviving son has had to be strong for the family, he has had to take over and 'do the things his dad should have done' because his dad could not cope with Matthew's death. Iris has, however, had to cope with the disruption to the family dynamics. She has offered an account of the effect on Matthew's brother and sister, and from this we can see that the effect on the wider family, and on her, has been far-reaching.

The extent to which it is appropriate to involve older siblings or to protect them is also a matter of concern:

> We were all under a strain and it showed. Each one of us put on a brave face (I can see through everybody). Sean assured me at one stage he was quite all right (aged nineteen now) but I could tell he had been crying. My daughter off-loaded to her friend who told her mother who told me. My eldest boy was away from home but got a bit 'woozy'. The school were very good to Ian, my youngest – just fifteen. I assured Ian his needs were important too. He had seen the brunt of Sean's illness, sharing a room with Sean. Ian coped well. He was attentive to Sean and good company. I was concerned about Ian and had wondered should he go and stop with my local friends (for Ian's sake). All nurses told me not to arrange that; Ian would cope better being involved with Sean, and they were right.
>
> (Charlotte)

Parents may attempt to protect siblings from witnessing the worst of the illness. Charlotte considered sending Ian away, after all he was seeing at close quarters what his brother was going through as they shared a room. However, the advice she was given, that Ian would cope better if he was involved, turned out to have been sound. If we think back to Chapter 1, we remember that Riches and Dawson (2000) also found that siblings sent away from home felt rejected and marginalized, and that however painful the sights at home may be, their security is there, and their imaginings of what is happening in their absence may be worse than the reality. To be there when a sibling dies may also allow closure in a way that being absent denies. Will siblings ever really be able to accept the death if they come home to find that their brother or sister has simply gone? However painful the process perhaps it has to be endured.

Lynn reflects on her attempts to protect her daughters from the extent of her grief:

> I struggled to protect Manda and Cindy from the full extent of my grief as it seemed a burden too big for them to bear and I know this hurt them very much. They felt as if they had lost their mother too, but

at the time I was so disabled with my grief I found it difficult to be a mother to my daughters. Our family has been fractured but we are still a family and gradually I was able to show my grief to the girls and gain a lot of comfort from them.

(Lynn)

It appears that Lynn's attempt to protect her daughters served to make them feel as though they had lost her as well as their brother, Simon Lynn says that she found it difficult to be a mother to her daughters and speaks of the 'fracturing' of the family.

Likewise, Denise refers to the 'emotional roller coaster' and its effect on her son Philip throughout his adolescence:

Philip was $12\frac{1}{2}$ when Laura was diagnosed and so has spent all of his teenage life in and out of hospital, dealing with the emotional roller coaster that families are on when you have a child with cancer.

(Denise)

It is worth noting that the phrase 'emotional roller coaster' has been used a number of times by different contributors. It is evocative of the tempestuous journey taken by the whole family when a young adult has cancer, and in the last passage it is clear that it affects all members of the family, including siblings.

Earlier in this chapter we considered the effect on Sue when she supported her younger son, Benjamin, through an illness after Alex's death from cancer. Her anxieties that he, too, might be seriously ill were happily unfounded, and it must be very rarely that siblings both develop cancerous conditions. However, this is what happened to Donald and Annie.

Fears for their own health as we have seen, may be one result of witnessing a sibling's battle with cancer but this anxiety is, thankfully, usually unfounded. However, very occasionally, the anxieties manifested by a sibling who has witnessed the cancer of a brother or sister may be well founded. When this happens, the previous experience of cancer in the family will affect the expectations and fears of the whole family as we see in Donald and Annie's account of their younger daughter Felicity's diagnosis of Hodgkin's disease. Their older daughter Donna had been diagnosed with acute lymphoblastic leukaemia six years earlier:

Felicity came to her mother with a lump on her neck in January 1997 and we attended our GP (Donna's had retired by now) within a few days. In two weeks she was seen by an ENT specialist. Something in my heart told me all was not well – the lump was not like a gland, it was like a rubbery nodular lump/lumps and quite big. Everyone kept saying it would be OK even our own GP but despite this we worried. Was it possible that she too had a cancer? We remembered asking the doctors in Glasgow after Donna was diagnosed if Felicity could get cancer as well and were reassured that the chance of two sisters in the same family having leukaemia were extremely rare if not unheard of . . . She had a biopsy done shortly after seeing the ENT consultant which confirmed Hodgkin's Disease. As always we didn't make a fuss, especially for Felicity's sake, but my heart was at my feet. I remember thinking; well at least it is not a brain tumour – given the choice! The treatment in comparison to leukaemia is much less aggressive and that seemed to lesson the gravity of the situation. Felicity was obviously doing her own comparisons and asked three questions from the consultant:–

1 Would it be two years' treatment?
2 Would she lose her hair?
3 Would she have to go to Glasgow?

As the answer was NO in every case the illness was no big problem in her eyes. She started 'chemo' (oral and IV) for about six months and things seemed to be going along fine until she developed another small lump on her neck during the October school holidays and unfortunately the disease had returned.

(Donald and Annie)

Donald and Annie say that their concern that Felicity might also develop cancer predated her illness. At the time of Donna's illness they even asked the specialist if Felicity might also be at risk. Whilst the answer was 'no', when Felicity's symptoms began their first thought and fear was that she too had cancer. It is interesting that in this instance, Felicity's experience of her sister's cancer, treatment and survival all appear to have prepared her for her own illness, particularly as her own prognosis and treatment regime appear to have been presented as less aggressive. Happily both daughters survived their different cancers and Donald and Annie continue their narrative by saying that Felicity had further intensive chemotherapy that appears to have been successful in curing her condition.

Balancing conflicting demands

So far, although the parents (mothers) have written them, the accounts have been presented largely in terms of the effects on their other children rather than reflecting directly the effect on them. However, we now come to accounts that demonstrate the effect on the parents (mothers) when trying to balance the needs of their sick children with the continuing needs of their other children.

Many of the previous accounts have been of older siblings, in a similar age group to their sick brother or sister, but younger children are also affected, though perhaps in different ways to older siblings. Candy's account of life as a single parent, having been recently widowed, demonstrates the difficulty of trying to meet the needs of all her children:

> My youngest daughter was only just 5 and my youngest son due to start secondary school. Because of the trauma of losing her father and obviously my emotional state Bethany wouldn't talk to anyone until she was nearly 7 and I had to keep 'abandoning' her so that I could be in London with Sianne. I used to spend two or three days with Sianne and then go home overnight to sort the others out and plan the next couple of days. I remember very clearly the terrible pain I felt having to leave either Sianne or Bethany when I knew how much they both needed me. I would sit on the train feeling so desperate and it used to take the one hour journey for me to be able to turn off from whichever one I had just had to leave.
>
> (Candy)

We see here that not only was Candy having to cope with terrible anxiety over Sianne's illness, she appears to be just as anxious, for different reasons about her younger daughter Bethany. Wherever she is she feels guilty and that she should be somewhere else. Bethany is too young to be taken on visits to Sianne, nor can she be left on her own. Again we see that single parenthood not only has an emotional impact, it has profound practical implications as no other parent was able to take responsibility for either visits to Sianne or the care of Bethany. Elizabeth, whose son Michael T died from osteosarcoma, makes a similar observation:

> I know one thing it is very hard when you are a single-parent who has a child with cancer and when you stay in hospital with your child while having treatment and seeing them going through pain and crying all the time. Plus when you've got another child who doesn't know what is going on it is very hard for one-parent to cope with.
>
> (Elizabeth)

The position both Elizabeth and Candy were in as single parents can be contrasted with the apparently easier (at least in practical terms) situation of Anne and her family. As she says:

> The effects on the family throughout his illness and after his death have been devastating and life will never be the same again. We also have three daughters. At the time of his death they were aged 24, 19, and just 12. My husband and I, both doctors knew something of the nature of his illness, maybe too much and keeping up the front of hope and cheerfulness for the children and each other was difficult . . . Most of his treatment was in the Hammersmith Hospital in London, a good three hour journey from our home. We travelled to and from the

hospital several times a week often together, too often alone. One parent with Chris, the other at home trying to keep life normal for our 11 year old.

(Anne)

This extract tends to suggest that being together lent enormous support to both parents, that they drew comfort from the knowledge that one of them was able to care for their youngest daughter, whenever necessary, and keep life as 'normal' as was possible. Interestingly Anne reflects on the lasting effect on her middle daughter:

> Our middle daughter will soon qualify as a doctor. She was the closest of the girls to Chris, and found it very hard to come to terms with his death. At university she co-founded an organisation called 'Marrow' which is a way to try and recruit bone marrow donors, working closely with the Anthony Nolan Trust. – 'Marrow' has now become active in several other universities in the U.K.

(Anne)

Although as Anne says, life will never be the same again after Christopher's death, and that her middle daughter who was closest to him found it very hard to come to terms with his death, we can see that she is trying to bring something positive from the experience – as George's younger brother did when he undertook the bike ride for charity. It may be that some action which pays tribute to the lost sibling acts as an important part of the grieving process, and may assist other family members in coming to terms with the loss. Such activity, and the additional anxiety it may cause is shown in Denise C's account of her son Ben's plan for a cycle ride in memory of his brother Alexander:

> Ben ... went through various plans of how to raise money for, in his case The Royal Marsden. One of these involved cycling from Newcastle to London, calling on every national cancer centre of excellence – i.e. leading cancer hospitals on the way until he reached the Royal Marsden. Fortunately for us, various obstacles couldn't be overcome and so instead a team from his school plus masters, 'relay-ran' from R.M.H London down to Devizes in Wiltshire over two days! What a feat. To us, it was a much safer option and one, which we could back up with support on route. However, the achievement and the event itself was so memorable and is still a very important stage in Ben's process of 'coming to terms' with the reality of Alexander's illness.

(Denise C)

Joyce's daughter Jill died at the age of 24 from osteosarcoma. Even though Jill's two sisters were old enough to be left while their mother was with her at the hospital during her treatment, Joyce expresses feelings of guilt for having left her other two daughters:

It was a stressful time for all the family. Jill was the middle daughter of three girls. Our whole life revolved around Jill. Fortunately the other two girls were old enough to take care of themselves, when we were away at Christie Hospital. I was constantly ringing them to keep them in touch. We felt guilty at times, because Jill took so much of our time, but the girls were very understanding.

(Joyce)

Joyce speaks of her daughters as being very 'understanding', as though she was away for work or even enjoying herself on holiday. She also says that their whole lives revolved around Jill. Whilst this does not denote any less love and concern for other children in the family, it still appears to lead to feelings of guilt.

Sue's family, which included Alex's younger brother, Benjamin and his younger sister, Natalie, had additional problems to contend with, here she reflects on the balance which had to be struck between their competing needs:

Benjamin found it very difficult to cope with the sight of his hitherto strong, tall, big brother reduced to a skeletal shape attached more or less non-stop to drips and lines. It was a novel experience for him to discover that Alex (always a little arrogant towards his younger siblings) now actually needed his companionship and looked forward to it. The two boys became closer than ever before, even though on the surface it was all about computer games!

With Natalie the situation was completely different. Five years earlier she had been diagnosed as suffering from borderline syndrome, a severe personality disorder, together with addiction problems. She needed endless amounts of (undivided) attention and her behaviour was often difficult, to say the least. That her brother was now equally in need of constant care and attention did not please her at all, and she became more withdrawn and problematic. Faced with the increased stress levels – especially as we were told that Alex would lose his leg – she cracked up and ended up in intensive care herself after an overdose.

Much to our intense regret, we simply could not cope any longer with these two very ill young adults and persuaded Natalie to accept the offer of a place in a psychiatric hospital, although we had always hoped to avoid that road. She spent the next four months on a locked ward, which was extremely distressing for us but at the same time a source of relief. Although it was almost impossible to rebuild a good relationship with her in that period, her absence from home made us aware of how much the rest of the family had been suffering. Freed from that terrible strain, everyone relaxed and the boys began to re-assess parent/child relationships, seeing perhaps for the first time the challenges we parents had been facing, found more comfort in their own relationship to each other, but developed more sympathy for their poor sick sister. As I was with Alex in hospital in England for two months towards the end of his life, the family was inevitably split up at a most difficult period. Natalie was back at school looking A levels in the face. Benjamin's girlfriend's father had just committed suicide . . . And their brother was far away, dying. But there seemed no other solution: Alex was happiest in England, with his friends around him, and anyway, I couldn't move him. So we had to compromise. Alex said he wanted to come home to die with his family all around him, and we did just that, so there was time for the other members of the family to be with him and say goodbye.

(Sue)

Sue and her family have clearly had to manage a number of significant problems, exacerbated by the geographical distance between Germany where they lived and England where Alex was treated. We also see the contrasting responses of Alex's brother and sister. His brother after the initial shock responded to Alex's new need of him and his companionship, while his sister, already living with mental health problems, found her condition was made much worse. We can only imagine the difficulty associated in deciding to persuade Natalie to enter a psychiatric hospital and indeed Sue uses the phrase 'intense regret', though under such circumstances it is hard to see what other decision could have been taken.

Reflections

The majority of narratives that have mentioned the presence of siblings in the family have addressed some sort of problem for the siblings arising as a result of the illness. It appears that whatever the age of the siblings, whether they are younger and need parental care or whether they are older and away from home, the effect of their brother or sister's illness can be far-reaching.

Much of the material from the narratives supports the literature considered in Chapter 1 (Spinetta *et al.* 1999; Riches and Dawson 2000), and the experiences of George's family. Siblings have experienced a range of problems and emotions, they have felt marginalized and isolated, and some have felt that they have 'lost' a parent as well as a brother or sister. They have also experienced fear and anxiety for their own health. However, in addition to documenting the problems from the siblings' perspective, we can see that these same problems cause the parents a considerable amount of additional distress.

Many of the narratives have indicated that parents feel guilt at having to divide their time and attention between their sick child and their other children. Whilst George's family appear to have managed this with minimal disruption to his younger brother, not all families have been so fortunate. The problem of 'where to be', and the feeling that wherever the parent is they are letting someone down, was expressed in a number of the narratives. This problem is exacerbated when the parent – usually the mother – is single handedly caring for the family.

Anderson's (2000) paper on responses to a death recognizes the importance of the bereavement process within the family. In most cases Anderson suggests that the acceptance of the loss occurs naturally over time, but in the case of siblings there may be many conflicting feelings to manage. Research conducted by Cain, Fast and Erikson (1964) shows that the death of a sibling can be mourned for many years and can put a strain on other relationships within the family. This may become a problem if feelings about the death have not been addressed or resolved at the time, for example if the surviving sibling has 'fallen out' with their brother or sister before their death this may lead to prolonged feelings of guilt (Anderson 2000).

It seems unavoidable that siblings will be affected, and that parents will take on the responsibility for the adverse effects. However, rather than parents feeling guilt at their inability to protect their other children from pain, or to be in two places at once, it is perhaps better to recognize that whatever strategy is adopted, there will always be an effect. It is worth noting that the reaction of one of the respondents to an article, which cited an academic expert commenting on how to manage siblings, left her feeling that the situation was not fully comprehended. She said:

> can't help feeling that it's fine for profs to say the obvious like 'do remember to love your other children while you are worrying yourself sick about the ill one' . . . the truth is, you just muddle through each day as best you can. No time, no energy, to read clever books about what to do and how to do it.
>
> (Sue)

It has never been the intention that this book should be one of the 'clever' ones referred to by Sue, or for it to offer advice on how the situation 'ought' to be managed. Rather, the intention of this book has been to document the lived experiences of those who have struggled, often failed, and sometimes succeeded in managing the impossible. To have access to such material can at least place individual struggles into a wider context that should act to relieve parents of guilt or feelings that they 'should' act in a particular way.

In relation to health professionals and others involved in the care of the young adult with cancer it is important that their awareness extends to siblings in the family. This is of particular importance within the community setting. Even if the professionals are not in a position to offer any material assistance, they should be aware of the potential problems and reassure parents that they are 'normal' under the circumstances. As Sloper (2000) observes, an important role for health professionals is to draw parents' attention to the needs of siblings and to ensure that information and support is available to them.

Garmezy (1985) has identified the importance of a positive support system in the family and in the siblings' wider network. Sloper (2000) comments on this study and suggests that such a support system might include: the provision of information in order to make sense of the situation; reassurance, which would help avert feelings of guilt; an understanding that fear and resentment are understandable responses; attention that makes siblings feel valued and helps to sustain self-esteem; support for siblings' own interests and opportunities to express their feelings.

In practical terms, for example in the case of single parents, other types of assistance may be offered. The *NHS Cancer Plan* (Department of Health 2000) emphasizes the importance of care within the community. If such care is to be of real assistance to parents, health professionals must be equipped with appropriate information to support parents in both emotional and practical ways with the care of their other children.

7 The financial implications for the family

George's story

I ended up not working. We have a reasonable family income and so were able to weather the costs of the illness but the costs are incredible. George had long periods in hospital, in Birmingham. We never left him in Birmingham on his own so not only did we have the journey costs up and down, we also had the cost of accommodation in Birmingham so we could be near him. As soon as the cancer was diagnosed I went on sick leave from work. We were very lucky in that my GP told me I must stay off work otherwise she would have two patients, not one patient to look after. And I couldn't possibly have worked anyway I felt so dreadful, though I did get a salary for quite a lot of the time. But eventually I did end up going through a period of, I can't remember how long, but several months with no salary. So my income, over a period of 4 or 5 years was definitely affected . . . either reduced pay or no pay for quite a lot of that period. I didn't go back to work either for at least 5 months after George had died because I became very ill myself, so again that was a period of no income. And when I did go back, I went back on reduced hours. So my earning capacity was reduced, at a time when I would have been thinking of increasing my working week from ³/₄ time to full-time once David was at secondary school. Instead I've actually ended up reducing my hours to half time. So several thousand pounds of my income, more than that, would have been lost. But in a sense it was really of no consequence in the overall scheme of things.

George, because he was a student, accepted that he was dependent upon us, and we accepted that it was his right and his entitlement. And it was the same situation that all his friends were in, they were students

depending on parents. But when he was home he didn't feel like a
student really, I think he felt like somebody unemployed so it felt very
important to get him benefits, so that he had some income that was not
from us, because he knew we were already incurring great costs simply
through having him ill. The income support rules are quite complex and
it was some time before George was eligible for benefits because it
seemed that if a university was holding a place for a sick student there
was a six month waiting period. Deep down I suspected that he would
never get back to Sheffield but it was desperately important for him to
have something to aim for and very important psychologically that his
departments were behaving as if this was just a temporary situation.
We couldn't possibly give up his place in order to claim benefits. We
also paid for his student accommodation for a period of 12 months after
his diagnosis, he had already found a student house to share with four
friends from his Halls and that was going to be theirs, I think from July.
And we actually paid George's share of the rent throughout the whole
of the academic year, which would have been George's second academic
year, just in case at any stage he felt that he could or wanted to go back,
so that was another cost . . . We were able to claim disability living
allowance for George, which he got about 6 months after the diagnosis.
I did all the paperwork for him as he found it very distressing to have to
admit that this situation might go on for a long time. So within 6 months
really of diagnosis George was in receipt of reasonable benefits, which
were an absolutely blessing because it was his money and it allowed
him to do whatever he liked. He could buy CDs, he could buy himself
a video machine, he could buy golf clubs, he was independent and he
could give himself treats without asking our permission, or without
them being things that he felt that we wouldn't necessarily approve of.
And he derived a lot of benefit, I think, from feeling that he did have an
independent income. I don't think we ever saw any of that for board
or lodging, we didn't ever ask, and it just made George feel a lot better
that he could, when he was well enough go away for weekends with
his friends. And buy . . . more expensive clothes to hide his very skinny
frame, and his sticky-out shoulder blades. And he did spend quite a lot
of money on clothes desperately trying to compensate for the loss of hair
and the paleness and the thinness, and we didn't mind that at all. So that
was good, it was good that George could actually do those things.

   I don't think he paid for very much of his own complementary
medicine out of his benefits. These were extremely expensive, although
he was very lucky in that we have a local cancer care charity where he
was entitled to massage, aromatherapy, counselling and hypnotherapy
and the Alexander Technique, that he didn't have to pay for. But in
addition to that he went to see a homeopath and an osteopath quite
often. Towards the end of his life he also went to the Bristol Cancer

Centre for a residential week which cost I think £500 or £600 but which he really enjoyed. We also went to see an alternative doctor in Leicester for a private consultation, a man who claimed to have success with diet and vitamins, that was very expensive. We all wished he was going to cure George. But I think George didn't really believe he would. But again that was another expensive consultation. The diet George adopted for a lot of the time, I think loosely called the 'Bristol Diet' was also very costly and required huge amounts of organic fruit and vegetables and vitamins and food supplements. It was also quite a time consuming as well expensive thing to do but it mattered desperately to George, and in a sense that was all that counted, we would go along with anything that gave him hope.

Wherever we could, whenever George was well enough, as a family we tried to do special and memorable things, we had several short holidays when he was ill. One was a holiday dictated by George's decision that he was going to cycle from Lands End to John O'Groats in the July before he died the following March. This was his answer to not having his lung removed. He was going to prove the doctors wrong by undertaking this physical feat and build himself up and build up his strength in his own way. That was extremely expensive because I by this stage was aware that George, short of a miracle, would not survive this illness. And so to make this bike ride possible, I just moved heaven and earth to find accommodation in lovely places, to pay the train fares and anything else that would make it a special event for George and for all of us really. So expense did not come into that at all, the whole thing cost a lot of money but it didn't matter. I think we probably bought George a new bike, and it didn't matter. Similarly a few months later in the October, 6 months before George died, again he wanted to do something special, he wanted to go to Dublin. By this time he was really beginning to get quite short of breath and tired extremely easily. We investigated every possible way of going to Dublin. We would have stayed in the most expensive hotel, but in fact in the end it was just not possible, he just wasn't well enough to make that journey. It was October half term and it was only realistic for him to go a short distance up to the Lake District. Most hotels were booked and I remember spending a whole day sitting on the phone determined that we would actually spend this October half term weekend in somewhere lovely because it was also Jonathan's 26th birthday. We ended up staying, there were six of us, in this hotel which we wouldn't normally even go to for a drink. We had every meal there, because George could only manage to walk down the grounds to the edge of the lake, and I think the whole bill for the weekend probably came to over a thousand pounds which is more than we would normally pay for a week's family holiday let alone a weekend. But again what mattered was to do it.

Another expense was Jonathan's wedding. He and his fiancée, Helen, decided, I think because they knew George may not be there in a year's time, that they should get married while George was well enough to attend the wedding. And again because we were doing this against the back-drop of George being in Birmingham for chemotherapy we didn't think of costs of outfits or of our contribution of the evening reception or anything like that, we just wanted it to be special. What we wanted was for everything to be as good as it possibly could be for everyone, and I'm very glad that we were in a position to do that. It must be very, very hard for those people who want to create special occasions and opportunities for the youngster who they know is going to have a short life and they actually can't afford it. Before George got ill, I used to really be quite doubtful I suppose about the benefits of those once in a lifetime trips, to Disney, but now I can see how much it matters. If not to the youngster, to the surviving families, that their child should have done during their life as many special things as can possibly be fitted in. And also it gives you something on the calendar that isn't a hospital outpatient appointment, isn't an x-ray, it's something on the calendar that is a contrast to all of those things. And so whenever we could, between treatments, George either on his own with friends when he was well enough, or with the family when he wasn't well enough used the time.

George and I used counselling I think to good effect for long periods probably for a couple of years. Both of us, I think often going weekly and the cost of that, for the two of us would be over £40 a week, this in addition to the free therapies he got from Cancer Care, which is our local cancer charity. Counselling was really quite a big cost and I guess it would have been available to us through the GP practice. In fact George was referred through the GP practice to the community psychiatric nurse but . . . the personalities were not right and George did not find it helpful. So buying psychotherapy meant that we were able to shop around and find somebody privately who George found extraordinarily helpful and who was really vital to George's coping strategies throughout the illness. But we were able to select because we were able and willing to pay. Another cost was Jonathan's fares up and down from London, which we were paying, I mean sometimes at a maximum cost on a Friday every two or three weeks. Later Helen came as well so we would quite often be spending £100 or more each fortnight on train fares. So there were all sorts of costs which just mounted up. But even so all the time we were also extremely grateful that he was receiving excellent and very, very expensive NHS care absolutely free of charge.

The financial implications when a child in the family is ill may be far-reaching. Costs, both expected and unexpected, may arise for a number of different reasons. Chapter 1 documents some of the causes of financial hardship when caring for a child with an illness or disability and many of these are manifested in George's story. As we see from George's mother's account, a parent – usually the mother – may have to give up work, and the cost of travel, accommodation and the provision of almost anything the sick child wants or needs can all act as a drain on family resources.

Financial dependency

The greatest concern for families caring for a young adult with cancer will be survival, and whilst the financial implications may add to the stress at the time, the long-term implications may not be addressed until after the illness is over. The life stage of the child when ill, may not at first sight seem relevant to the financial impact, after all such issues would seem to apply at any age, but Sue links life stage and financial problems closely:

> Most young people will still be financially dependent on their parents, who may be struggling to meet mortgage repayments and other siblings in further education, training or school.
>
> This may well be the most challenging time financially and cause more problems than with younger children. Yet we discovered that we were not eligible for much help, nor was the situation perceived to be possibly problematic. Whilst younger children are often (and rightly) on the receiving end of charity handouts, the spotty, rebellious teenager misses out!
>
> We are not strapped for cash, yet we soon felt the pinch as terminal disease can take a long time. Many of the items we needed for Alex were not completely covered by our health insurance (in Germany) and we had to pay for some things out of our own pocket. Much money was lost on airfares that we had to cancel, paying for rent for accommodation nobody was using (although the university did its utmost to reduce this to a minimum), fetching belongings etc. from England, not to mention the little treats that we wanted to give Alex in an attempt to make his life more pleasurable. During the last three months I had to give up work completely in order to be with Alex in England and then look after him at home, so there was another reduction in income (no disability living allowance in Alex's case here). Funeral costs were high, even though we did nearly everything ourselves, and as a young student does not normally have any assets to bequeath to his relatives, there was no inheritance to offset the expense. At the same time we were paying maintenance for Natalie to live in her own flat. Now, we are in a position to sort this out (we cashed in a life insurance), but others families might not be so

fortunate. Hearing well-meaning friends advising me shortly after Alex's death to go 'on a damn good holiday for a month with the family', made me wonder if they appreciated the financial struggle that could be involved.

(Sue)

A number of issues are raised here. Whilst as Sue says she and her family were 'not strapped for cash', the financial impact has still been difficult to manage. The lack of benefits, the loss of income whilst caring for Alex, and no inheritance to cover funeral costs as would usually be the case with an older relative. As with George's family, (unused) university accommodation was also paid for. But to add insult to injury, Sue feels that few people appreciated the degree of financial sacrifice involved, and that holidaying for a month with the family was simply not an option.

These sentiments are echoed by Brenda who reflects on the expense incurred by allowing Miles to pursue attempts at finding 'cures' and keeping in touch with his friends, perhaps the only things he could do to attempt to take control of his life:

The amount of money Miles was spending on telephone and alternative medicines. Miles was doing a lot of research into his illness before he became too ill to care. He was determined to try every alternative 'cure' possible. Whilst this kept him motivated and positive I do think that a few people take advantage of this and we watched our son send hundreds of pounds to a doctor in America in return for boxes of natural pills and medicines which were supposed to give him vitamins and supplements to fight cancer. If he ever detected our criticism or concern that he was being duped he would get angry with us for being negative. It became easier just to let him send off the money even though I was worried that he was getting into debt. The amount of phones calls he made also became a source of worry. Sometimes he would be on the phone all day long as this was a good way of passing his long days of inactivity. I think he began to lose all consideration of mundane matters like money and became consumed with the battle of survival. In many ways he became childish with his frustration with the constraints of his illness. Sometimes, he would yell at us to stop fussing around him, that he had once been self-sufficient. He would then feel guilty and I would curse that we were all trapped in this 'no win' situation . . . Taking him [to hospital] was really a 'two man' job . . . After some time we made friends with the hospital doorman who would take over the parking of our car for us. However we would have to give a large tip and we've anxiously seen our savings deplete. The petrol to and from London was expensive on top of everything else.

(Brenda)

When coupled with the travelling expenses to and from the hospital and the attendant expenses of tipping (we saw in Chapter 2 how difficult it was for Miles's parents to manage the hospital visits as he refused to use a wheelchair) we can see that financial issues became a source of contention, which when added to the concern over his health must have made family life very problematic. Once again life stage is a factor. Miles saw his parents' attempts to guide him as interference, yet his need to assert his independence in making unwise choices are issues unlikely to be experienced by other age groups. He was also, it appears, no longer financially independent thus the tension between his reluctant need for dependency, his quest for autonomy and his parents' concern over his use of resources must all have combined to result in a situation even more fraught.

The plight of Candy, a single widowed parent, also highlights the financial problems encountered when caring for a child with cancer:

> I also was struggling financially because I only have widowed mothers' allowance and was so grateful for the help I received from some cancer charities. I remember so well standing in the hospital garden late at night staring up at the stars begging for someone or something to help me, but it never came.
>
> (Candy)

While it seems that Candy did receive some financial assistance, it also appears that this was insufficient to alleviate her problems.

The need to provide the young adult with things to look forward to and to plan for may conflict with a wish to be able to give up work in order to be with the sick child. We can see from Sue B's account that she struggled with just such conflicting emotions and had to juggle a number of cross-cutting agendas:

> Strange feelings today. A couple of times I've felt elated as I think of the future and what we can do or where Paul could go. Seems strange. Only a few days [ago] the future was the one thing I would not allow to enter my head. I know the future, especially the next few months will probably be very difficult – how can we keep Paul's positive spirit working? – The boredom and frustration must be dealt with. I am also realising that tension can creep in and I must not allow my selfish reactions to take hold. Mom and dad will need support too. I must not be a burden. I have considered leaving work, resigning my post and many other alternatives but I now have one ambition – to save enough for Paul to go to Iceland. I need my money for that. I'm afraid school will have to suffer but as little as possible. I shall get organised.
>
> (Sue B)

Lynn recounts the additional costs of a holiday, rendered much more expensive because of Simon R's condition:

It was a wonderful holiday and considering the strain we were all under it went very smoothly. Because of Simon's condition the insurance cover cost a small fortune but we had no problems with the flights . . .

(Lynn)

Although it is clear that the costs were considerable, the value of the holiday for the whole family is incalculable. The memories that abide after the death make the cost a secondary factor. Lynn also mentions an additional and unexpected related expense in the following extract:

Jessie our cat died on the 25th October – she had been diagnosed with bowel cancer four months previously. It was a difficult decision to let her go as the correlation between her and Simon was too close for comfort, the kindest thing to do when she was diagnosed was euthanasia but Simon loved her lots, she had been with him all his life (she was 20 years old – which is bloody old for a cat) and as he said, 'why put her down? – I've got cancer will you put me down?' So we spent a fortune keeping her alive and fairly healthy for his sake – it was cruel, but we had no choice. Simon saw himself in her and almost seemed to be waiting for her demise as a measure of his time. Simon sobbed like a baby when she died and I knew then that he saw his approaching departure.

(Lynn)

Again it is clear that all other considerations are secondary to making the remaining time better in whatever way that can be managed, in this case keeping alive an elderly and ailing cat, but there must be a myriad of other decisions made daily that all have a financial impact on the family.

The struggle with bureaucracy

Not only are financial problems difficult to manage, they may be made worse by an inadequate knowledge of the very complex benefits system. It is not always clear to parents – and sometimes it seems to professionals – what young adults are entitled to in their own right in terms of benefits or what the family may be able to claim to care for them. Part of the problem seems to be that at this life stage the young adult's status as a student, or as a member of the labour force without enough National Insurance (NI) contributions, makes such calculations problematic. Quite apart from the financial implications of such matters, the struggles with bureaucracy may be exceedingly stressful as we can see in the following two accounts:

Whilst trying to deal with the physical and emotional sides of the illness we also had to fight the bureaucracy of the County Council and the Government.

I rang the Education Department as soon as possible after the New Year to advise them of the situation. They said that as Tim had dropped out the whole of his grant would have to be reassessed. We assumed that as he had completed a term that the reassessment would be from January – this proved to be wrong. The grant was looked into for the whole year and both Tim and his brother received demands to repay the grant they had spent in the Christmas term. The reassessment showed that due to the fact Tim had dropped out, they could not receive any grant for that academic year. We lodged an appeal against the decision as the money had been spent in good faith and we did not see why we should be penalised because of Tim's illness. This did not stop them sending out final summonses and threats of court action whilst the appeal was being considered.

We also tried to enlist the help of our MP over the problem, he was of some help in pushing our cause and we did win our appeal after his intervention. However when further problems developed our MP would only quote Government documents at us.

As Timothy had no means of support or income we decided to apply for incapacity benefit. This was refused on the grounds that he had not paid enough NI contributions. We then applied for income support but were refused on the grounds that students could not claim income support because they were getting a grant. We then went back to LCC and discussed the situation with them, however as far as they are concerned Tim was no longer a student and could not therefore receive a grant.

We wrote to our MP again on the subject and he sent us documentation showing that the local council can continue to pay grants under exceptional circumstances such as severe illness. We went back to LCC who advised us that they only administer grants on behalf of the government and they had been advised that in our case Tim was no longer a student and a discretionary grant could not be paid.

We then went back to the DSS and decided to appeal against their decision to refuse to pay income support. Armed with all the information we could gather, and a letter kindly produced by Reading University saying Tim had abandoned his course permanently, we won our appeal. (The university did add later that the letter did not preclude Tim from finishing his course if he ever wanted to return. Part of the argument from the DSS was that you had to abandon your course permanently with no intention of returning). Tim then received income support for the rest of the period of his illness. Whilst we could have afforded to support Tim during his illness he was feeling depressed that his illness was costing us money, he was having to ask for every penny he wanted to spend and had no independent means.

(Jeremy and Lesley)

We can only imagine the additional stress that Jeremy and Lesley endured trying to claim what was, after all their rights. However, the financial impact is only part of the issue, as Jeremy and Lesley say, their son's morale, which was lowered in any case by being ill, needed to be boosted. He was depressed by the fact he was costing them money, and, even though they were in the fortunate financial position to be able to support him, it was demoralizing to have to ask for every penny he spent to be given to him.

We see that similar frustrations were encountered by Sue B when Paul was trying to claim benefit:

> The frustrations came through the post. The DHSS sent a stupid letter asking why he'd claimed since November 30th and only informed them on 3.1.91. Said they'll have to reconsider his claim. No cheque has arrived. The taxman has caught up with him. Disappointing but inevitable. I am annoyed for Paul's sake but angry that we live in a society that is as inefficient as this that there is little communication between departments. I don't know whether to go up and complain – write or leave it to Paul. I'll ask him. Whatever would happen if he was living alone – trying to keep well, pay rent and they stop his money through their inadequacies. It makes my blood boil.
>
> (Sue B)

Here there is recognition by Sue B that although Paul is an 'adult' the chances of him dealing successfully with this system without parental help is minimal. While he was eventually awarded benefits of £47 per week, this had to be fought for, and is still demonstrably not enough for him to be 'independent'.

Christine, as a single parent on a relatively low income was not in such a fortunate position, so her struggles with bureaucracy were even more stressful and their outcome even more vital for her ability to manage the illness and its financial implications.

> 'Cause I wasn't actually on benefits, so, yeah it was difficult. But Tony got DLA [Disability Living Allowance] so that was all right. But I found it, I just found all of it so stressful. I felt like nobody understood. 'Cause even when I was on the phone, I seemed to be shouting at everybody all the time. I know I was stressed, but I was shouting, and I wrote to MPs, and I was just so mad. Even with the Benefit Agency, I mean, you know, you have to wait like, they don't realise that you haven't got any money . . . 'Cause you are claiming for so many, you have to fill so many forms in. I mean, I didn't have the time to be honest. I didn't have the time to fill the forms in. You had to fill one for income support, one for disability living allowance, one for incapacity, council tax benefit. And all these people writing to you saying

'you've not filled this in, and you've not filled that in' and I was waiting to hear from them. I mean, it took them about, I think it took them about three months to sort the claim out. In the end they did actually give me arrears, but in that time it was like letters, which, you know I was backwards and forwards to the hospital and everything. I mean it's like invalid care allowance, I mean, really that is a bad benefit if you are a single parent because you only get £10 a week anyway, but the hassle you got for actually filling the forms . . . 'cause if you're a single parent you actually get a top-up on your child benefit but because, if you get invalidity care allowance they take that benefit off you, single parent benefit off you. So it's like sending my book back to child benefit, you know, all these things going around, and you've got this child who's terminally ill. I mean at the end of the day, you know, you just felt like, in the end I used to just get on the phone, and you're on the phone, and you get through and you have to explain it to people, then you'd have to say it all over again, you know. And then they didn't know what to do. And then they'd transfer you to somebody else. And in the end I just got the supervisor, I just went straight through to them and thought you know. I found that so hard because it's not a nice thing, you go through it all, and people, you know you could tell they were quite upset anyway. But yeah, the benefit system was horrendous . . . at home, say for the first week after the treatment he was really poorly, he was in bed and everything, and things. But after that he seemed to get himself up a bit. We used to go out a lot, if he was fine, if he wanted to go out we'd just go. And I mean, without having any money I just couldn't have done that, you know. And I made sure, 'cause I'm quite into healthy eating, and I was getting all these books . . . I did a course on complementary medicine, but it was only like a basic one. But when he was in hospital I got books and was reading what to give him to eat and, he had everything. If I thought it was doing him any good, fruit or vitamins and things, I gave it to him . . . I used to stock the fridge up with anything that he just fancied, you know. He used to like strawberries at one time, so I used to always get strawberries. It was everything he wanted. He had certain crazes on different foods and then sometimes he didn't. Especially, when they are on chemotherapy they are prone to infections as well, so you know, I had to be careful of all the sell by dates on different things, I used to buy it, used to throw it away . . . there was certain foods he liked, I can't remember them now . . . Anything he wanted he could have. I mean, and a lot of it was DLA, I mean without that I couldn't have managed, no way. Even just going to Blackpool. I mean my sister just spent an absolute fortune.

(Christine)

This extensive extract from Christine's narrative has been included not only because she lists a number of different causes of financial concern, but also because of the way in which it communicates the distress she felt. The struggles with the Benefits Agency, her frustration over the forms, the lack of assistance she received, the amount of time she had to wait to hear from them, the expense of special food and trips out. All these had to be managed whilst she also had to live with the knowledge that her son might be terminally ill. In her own words 'I felt like nobody understood'. So here again we see a single parent struggling not only with financial hardship to provide her child with anything that would make his life more pleasant, it is also clear that she encountered considerable problems in claiming her entitlement to benefit from an apparently bureaucratic system.

Reflections

There is no doubt that illness is expensive. This has already been established through the literature referred to in the first chapter of this book (Baldwin 1985; Bone and Meltzer 1989; Bennett and Abrahams 1994; Beresford 1995; Dobson and Middleton 1998; Corden *et al.* 2001). It is endorsed by George's story and borne out by the narratives. The expenses are many and varied, and may leave the family in debt, or with depleted savings, long after the illness is over. The situation is exacerbated in this age group by a number of factors. First, young adults have a degree of autonomy, but little money of their own with which to finance the lifestyle they may try to maintain. Second, if they are students they may have to choose between giving up their studies and claiming Benefit, and parents such as George's may struggle to support them financially and relinquish benefit for the sake of morale and the belief that they will return to their studies. Third, treats, trips and holidays may all be an important need for the whole family, but perhaps at this life stage expectations of what a treat might consist of are more expensive. Fourth, many young people may be attracted by alternative therapies and decide to pursue these in addition to their orthodox treatments; such therapies are, however, extremely expensive and it is unlikely that young adults will have the independent means through which to finance them.

Despite this list of costs, it is clear that financial issues are of secondary importance. They may cause problems, and may have lasting effects, but they pale into insignificance when compared to the possible loss of a child. Indeed financial concerns may be almost impossible to articulate at the time for fear that somehow a 'price' is being put on the illness. Therefore they are put to one side to worry about later. Yet if the 'later' is after the death of a son or daughter, the additional financial concerns must make the bereavement even more stressful with the addition of practical problems.

Some of the accounts of financial difficulties presented in this chapter relate to problems in both understanding and accessing statutory entitlements. However, as some of the accounts may relate to a period when benefits were awarded under a different system, not all the experiences may be relevant to current regulations, which are discussed at the end of this chapter. Nevertheless, many of the issues are still relevant and difficulties in gathering useful and accurate information and succeeding in claiming benefit entitlements remain the same whatever the detail of the claim.

There appear to be particular problems relating to students whose benefit entitlements are complex and often unclear to parents and professionals alike. As a social worker, George's mother was in a better position than most to know what his entitlements were, but she still struggled with the apparent need for George to withdraw from university before he was entitled to claim benefit. Coxon (2001: 10) supports this assumption in a feature in *Guardian Education*. She says that in order to claim benefit for the first six months of an illness, a student would have to withdraw from university. As the subheading says 'You desperately want to finish your course, but you fall ill. Then to cap it all, you discover that for 28 long weeks you will get no financial help from the State at all'. Students who are diagnosed with cancer may well wish to retain their student status in the belief that they will return to their studies after the illness is over. Many never recover sufficiently to return to university, and some die before they complete their degrees as George did. Yet they have to believe that return to student life is a possibility and given the importance of identity as we saw in Chapter 1, to retain that identity as a student when all others are being stripped away by illness is of fundamental importance. Additionally the significance of those around them, both in the family and the medical profession, making a statement in the belief of their recovery, is of vital importance, and the fact that George's parents continued to pay for accommodation he never used, kept his spirits up and helped him to believe he could recover. He also retained his student status – an important part of his identity.

The *NHS Cancer Plan* (Department of Health 2000) as discussed in the first chapter has as part of its agenda the commitment to sustain the care of patients with cancer in the community. Yet it is difficult to see how this can be managed without adequate benefits, which are accessible, easy to claim and readily known at a time when tussles with bureaucracy must appear intolerable. However, to retain student status under most circumstances will mean no entitlement to benefit.

There are exceptions to this regulation, which are based on a student being awarded status as a 'disabled student', and thus being able to claim Income Support. This can be achieved through two means – either by the student being declared unfit for work for 28 weeks; or claiming Disability Living Allowance either as a result of having a certain degree of care or supervision needs, or mobility difficulties, for three months or being issued with a DS1500 through the recommendation of a medical practitioner. However, the issue of a DS1500 is based on a declaration that the young person is not likely to live for more than six months. The need to retain student status may be important, but the need to believe in recovery is even more important, therefore the DS1500 route, even if applicable, may be unacceptable to many parents and students alike – it is after all an admission of the loss of any hope. Even if a student can claim Disability Living Allowance under the normal three-month qualifying period rule, it may take several months to process. Only when classified as a 'disabled' student can an Income Support claim be made and even then, as it is a means tested benefit, a student, without income or savings may still not qualify. This is because the student loan facility is counted as 'income', and this is the case even if a student has chosen not to take out a student loan. While medical practitioners can facilitate the process of a claim for benefits, they cannot circumvent the procedural routes and are thus limited in their ability to assist a student to qualify for financial help via the benefits system.

The situation relating to students as described here is only accurate at the time of publication, and successive governments may implement policy changes. However, the main principles remain the same even though the details may change across time. That is, that the system is complex and difficult to manage for both students and non-students and that accurate and helpful information is hard to find. The implications for professionals are obvious; they need to have a clear understanding of benefits and entitlements and must be in a position to assist parents in claiming them. We have seen the struggles with form filling and bureaucracy endured by parents, if this burden is alleviated at least one anxiety will be lifted. This would appear to be of particular importance in relation to single parents who may struggle financially under the best of circumstances and if they are forced to give up work the expense of the illness may become prohibitive.

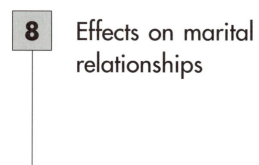

8 Effects on marital relationships

George's story

It appears to me that from the moment of George's diagnosis until the day he died nothing else really mattered to me. Apart from I suppose the emotional survival of Jonathan and David, but George's well-being and George's fight for survival, how he felt, how he was coping, what he was feeling were absolutely essential for every waking moment. I know I had much more difficulty sleeping than Geoff did. I don't think I slept more than an hour at a time, for about 4 years. I would fall asleep, then I would wake up with a racing heart being in an absolute state of panic . . . knowing exactly why I was in a panic the minute I hit consciousness and this would just go on throughout the night. The only peace I really got I think was when I was with George and doing something for him or providing something for him that I felt or hoped made him feel better. Whether it was doing the Guardian *crossword in bed or buying a new CD that he wanted, or making a special meal if he would eat, or buying bits of things that might interest him. Whatever it was, I really only I think had any peace when I could actually be doing something for George, which was an enormous burden for him. I am absolutely sure that he and I knew what one another was thinking without speaking. And it felt to me as if not only was I actually feeling my own pain but I was also feeling George's pain. I could tangibly feel his physical pain when he was unwell or when he was sick and I could feel his emotional pain. I'm not sure that that's the way I would be affected by the other two boys, or whether it was something peculiar to the relationship between myself and George. I'm sure that Geoff had a much healthier ability to cope with the pain of it all than I did. Geoff certainly could continue to work in a way that I couldn't have done, although I did work for some periods during George's illness. Geoff always had a briefcase with him so whenever we were waiting for the result of biopsies or waiting for ward rounds or sitting by George's hospital bed or waiting at home for him when he was well enough to get up and come downstairs, Geoff could always work in a way that I couldn't. I could only really do things that I felt were going to make George in the short term or the long-term feel better . . . Geoff and I did share tasks between us though. George often slept or did very little during the day-time and then became quite nocturnal, especially during the times when he was at his poorliest. And quite often he would really be at his liveliest at 11, or midnight and quite often would say to me, 'mum can we have a talk?' And I think this happened more and more during the night for the last 12 months before he died. And I remember being up with him sometimes till 5 in the morning just listening while he talked about his feelings about life, his feelings about his illness about all sorts of philosophical issues while he tried to work out for himself what his illness meant. And however tired I was I could always stay for as long as George needed to talk. Geoff couldn't, by midnight he was shattered. Because he continued working, he hadn't had any time off work and if he did like the times in Birmingham he was always making phone calls or sending mail or posting things up and down or even driving up and down so that he could keep his workload going. But whatever George needed, however unreasonable or whatever it was I could always find the energy to meet those needs. What I couldn't do and what Geoff did was I couldn't bear to go to any of the reviews in Birmingham which were three monthly, from the end of the first set of chemotherapy throughout George's illness, when there was no active treatment there was always check-ups that involved CT scans, often MRI scans and X-rays in Birmingham and I couldn't go to those. I just knew that my level of anxiety was so high I couldn't actually tolerate being there and George would have been acutely aware as to how I felt. I don't know how Geoff felt, I guess he felt pretty awful, but however he felt he was able to hide it from George. So the check-ups which gave George the diagnosis of lung secondaries and a recurrence of those secondaries were given to Geoff and to George with me having the news on the phone. I also didn't go down to Birmingham on the very first occasion until I had about 24 hours at home to compose myself. So when George came back from Sheffield and went straight down to Birmingham within 48 hours I stayed at home, just to try to get my head straight, so I could try to cope with what lay ahead. Geoff didn't do that . . . I know that Geoff had to cope with quite difficult behaviour from George on several of those check-ups. I know that one time, I think when George was given the diagnosis of lung secondaries, he threw his x-rays, his medical notes* around the consultant's office and then kicked parking cones all around the car park and ranted and raved in a way that you don't normally see in hospital corridors. And I don't know how Geoff coped with that. I don't think I would have been able to cope with it really. Though we've been married a long time, we have different strengths, I think we respected that there were some things that one of us could do that the other one couldn't do, and we didn't question that, we just sorted it out between us. Most of the liaison with health professionals and complementary practitioners I did because that was my job. As a hospital social worker I knew how to access information and services within health and Geoff didn't and he left that to me. We didn't talk very much about our feelings to one another, there didn't seem to be a lot of point we were in this dreadful place that we had to get through somehow for the sake of the whole family and we did it in different ways. But I think we had a mutual respect for our different ways of doing things. It did become difficult at the end when I needed to spend all my time with George after he became iller and Geoff tried to take on the domestic tasks. He found that really quite difficult the shopping and the preparing of meals, we had a lot of help with that from friends. But when Geoff took on the domestic role, which was probably for a period of I suppose no more than 6 to 8 weeks so that I could totally give George the emotional and personal support that he needed, that was a difficult time. But I think we know what one another are thinking and feeling without having to talk about it. Geoff doesn't feel that it helps to talk about his feelings, I do, but I have a big network of friends with whom I can talk. And also I went to counselling for about 2 years. Because I think one of the big gender differences between Geoff and I was that Geoff always believed that until the worst happened you must believe the best. And I think that I believed really very strongly, through most of George's illness that he wasn't going to survive and I needed a safe place where I could talk about the way that I'd been feeling. And I did that through counselling, which is something that Geoff would never have thought to do, which allowed me an escape and a person to speak to who wasn't in any other way involved with the situation. I felt I had to protect everybody who was close to George from the negative feelings that I had. That was really quite hard . . . especially once the lung secondaries had appeared because I'd got much more medical experience than Geoff and I knew that things were now very dire indeed in a way that Geoff couldn't or wouldn't acknowledge. In terms of the different ways Geoff and I coped with George's illness, there was the fact that I actually went for paid counselling, for hypnotherapy through our local Cancer Charity and took anti depressants and at times beta blockers when we were waiting for the results of one of George's reviews or waiting for him to come out of operating theatres. Geoff did none of those things, he didn't

have any medication and he didn't have any counselling to help him
through it all. He was aware that I found them helpful but he didn't feel
that they were of any value for him.

Chapter 1 establishes, largely through the work of Rosenblatt (2000a, 2000b), that men and women grieve differently. It is also clear that illness in the family is differentially experienced both in practical terms and in its emotional impact (Brannen *et al.* 1994). George's mother's account suggests that she and her husband did indeed implement different coping mechanisms and approaches to George's illness. However it appears that in this instance George's parents, while responding differently, complemented one another, each adopting a different role in relation to George, the management of his illness and the practicalities of family life. However, rather than these different roles dividing the couple and the family it seems that they were mutually supportive and reflective of an unstated understanding of each other's needs.

The majority of the respondents whose stories are told in this book were married or had partners. Most of the narratives were written by mothers, and in these the husband/partner remains a shadowy figure in the background, mentioned only in passing. Where the male partner is referred to in some detail it is usually with reference to problems in the relationship exacerbated by the impact of the illness.

An awareness of the danger in which a marriage can be placed is shown in the following extract. However, while Mary, whose daughter Nicola died from malignant melanoma, does not say that she and her husband are having marital problems she does acknowledge the need for communication if the marriage is to survive:

> Perhaps one of the most important things for parents is to be supported as a couple – if they are living together. Although I was aware of the fact that the tragedy of a child's illness or a child's death is a frequent cause of parental separation, I thought that the common unspoken bond of the pain of the tragedy was sufficient. But it isn't. Parents must need support in communicating if the marriage is to continue. In such a painful situation, both during the progress of the cancer (which these days may be over many years) and afterwards in the bereavement many parents must need support in communicating their feelings to each other.
>
> (Mary)

The importance of communication is interesting here. George's mother says that the communication between her and Geoff was 'unspoken', that they had been married for so long each knew what the other's strengths and limitations were and that each responded accordingly without having to articulate their needs.

In another example of a marriage that has survived the death of a child, Anne's account tells us of the importance of the relationship to both her and her husband. However, she also acknowledges that he cannot talk about his feelings:

> For me personally as his mother the pain of watching your child suffer physically, mentally and emotionally is torture. His death was a relief to us all after watching him suffer so much. For so long the image of his last days fighting for breath will always be me . . . Now 3 years on our grief is still very deep but obviously less acute. We talk about him naturally and the things he did, good and bad, as if he is just away from home. Christmas, New Year, Easter are all difficult times and we are always aware of his last days on these occasions, when he was so ill and trying so hard not to be . . . My husband and I reaffirm our love often – a desperate need to cling on to each other, but he can't talk about his feelings which I have to respect . . . I am depressed more than ever (I have suffered depression life-long) and now have a diagnosis of M.E. The only thing to keep me going is the thought that my daughter needs me, otherwise what is the point of anything . . . I am on the local committee for Leukaemia Research Fund. I have become a bereavement counsellor for Cruse, but I don't have the energy for much else. My husband works full-time but also seems to lack drive and energy he once had.
>
> (Anne)

Denise C likewise reflects on the gendered division of labour and differentiated response which exists between her and her husband Phil:

> an immediate agreement of sharing all the trauma as equal partners was a natural outcome, creating an even more special bond between the two of us. Neither of us felt that we stood alone any more, on any issue to be faced . . . A few specific consultations I could not face, so Phil always was willing to be brave and accompany Alexander, thus lightening my burden. Again an agreed and shared responsibility. Phil and I used the time on our own to discuss how best we could handle whatever lay ahead in practical terms but we never revealed to each other how we really felt inside for fear of upsetting emotions even more. I wanted to share my despair but knew that talking freely might interfere with all the 'positive' aspects that we shared. Therefore I tried to keep my 'crying time' till I was alone . . . Phil was never afraid to cry a little but I always felt there was more 'bottled up' which he wouldn't or maybe couldn't release . . . Phil keeps a lot to himself. He has always been a very private person, I can usually sense when he is feeling down but pray that he could tell me more. I still feel he won't, in order to protect

my emotions. Sometimes I wish I could tell him how I am. I hint at it but never reveal the true depth.

(Denise C)

Denise C's account has much in common with both George's story and Anne's in that both Anne's husband and George's father were less able to talk about their feelings than were their wives. Despite these differences, it seems that the bond between Anne and her husband and between Denise C and Phil remains strong – as it has with George's parents – the differences being accepted, each partner adopting a different but equally valued role. It seems significant that although Denise C says that she feels that her husband Phil cannot be as open with her as she would like, she also acknowledges that she cannot communicate with him the true extent of her pain. Here it seems are two people who care about each other very deeply and who are each afraid to cause the other additional pain by emotionally 'offloading' their own. So, their partnership does not appear to have been damaged by their loss and later in her narrative Denise C says that she feels their lives have an added dimension as a result of their experience and that they are stronger people as a result.

However, in contrast, the following extract addresses the issue of a marital relationship in crisis:

What has losing Susan done to me and Brian? I'll have to put things down as I remember. I was sedated most of the time before she died. I went to bed crying knowing it could be Susan's last day. Also from the hospice, I came home crying. The phone when Susan lived in Germany was used a lot. My bills were sometimes £150. After the 5/6/96 I can't remember living (that's the truth) between 5/6/96 to when we cremated Susan 13/6/96 her birthday ... We went out each day, I don't know where, Blackpool, walked along the prom. Bumped into people (dazed), everyone laughing, enjoying themselves. I felt like screaming Susan's dead. I don't know whether I cooked, cleaned or even showered ... I cried for three months in the car and in the bus whenever I passed the hospice ... [I] cried all the way home. I dreaded going home because I would always RING SUSAN at once ... I saw daffodils in the garden. First time someone said Christmas '99 'you look better than you did 1½ years ago'. I didn't know I looked ill. I lost two stones. At first you feel physically sick, palpitations. I would not get out of bed one week. Went to doctors got pills. I didn't know how would have got through. Cry at a drop of a hat. Names, places, shopping all hurt. Brian could not leave me at all on my own, I would PANIC. One afternoon I was on my own and I cried, cried till I was exhausted. I still cry now. First year seemed easy, still awful [but] I was able to say 'this time last year [I] was doing this and that'. Second year was 'is it true?' dreaming she would come back. Third year, well you are realising she will not come back. HELP. As for Brian and I, well our marriage is hanging on by a thread, it wasn't that good before, but I had Susan there for me. THAT'S WHAT I MISS.

(Jean)

Despite the fact that the extract begins by asking the question 'what has losing Susan done to me and Brian?' and ends with a reflection on the fragility of the marriage, most of this section of the narrative is about the pain Jean feels. It seems that a marriage described as 'not that good before' has only suffered as a result of the pain and loss. Though Jean says that at one stage her husband could not leave her or she would panic, this need does not seem to have been translated into a mutually sustaining relationship as she tells us that her marriage is hanging by a thread. It may be that whatever characteristics or underlying problems a marriage has prior to the illness are exacerbated by it.

In an account of the failure of a marriage Carol tells us that her husband found a new partner after their daughter's death.

Following Sara's death, my husband found another partner and this ended our marriage. I now work in bereavement for a cancer care service. I have come to realise that we all grieve differently, especially parents, and often in one family. A few months after Sara died, my husband accused me of 'seeing' him again – pointing out that I hadn't for a long time. I took this on board, along with all the other guilt, but after we'd separated, I realised that this hadn't been altogether true. He was an egotistical man with a need for attention and he'd found this elsewhere with a young woman of Sara's age – he needed to blame me of course: it eased his own conscience. I found myself on the other side of the county in a country cottage, with no job and little money. I still bear the financial scars, but the more livid ones are ever present, and grief being what it is, always waiting to be re-opened.

And now? I have a new life, a different one certainly from the one I envisaged in October 1994. The Millennium was hard, cruelly so. Sara should have been with us. I would have liked her to meet Simon who has given me back my belief that there <u>can</u> be hope. I trust him implicitly. Perhaps it's <u>change</u> in the end which helps most, even change that seems small: that, and time, and courage.

(Carol)

Carol acknowledges that people grieve differently and that when this happens in a family – for example when two partners grieve differently – it can be the source of conflict. This would concur with the discussion of the literature in the first chapter. However, Carol suggests that this explanation is too simplistic, and that her ex-husband's egotism coupled with his need for attention was at least in part responsible for their separation. Thus again we see that the pre-existing relationship is crucial.

The following extract also reflects on the difference between partners. Again it is lengthy and many issues are addressed but we see some resonance with the experiences already expressed:

My dear Mike is plodding on. He was very emotional on New Year's Eve – more than I've known before. Yesterday and today he's very quiet and wrapped up in his own world. I wish he'd express his feelings. Everyone was great at work, mom and dad let me cry it out, Jacqui said I mustn't let Paul see me like this, Marg [Sue B.'s sister] was great but said I had to get a grip and Mike told me I needed to change my attitude!! This last one hurt but was true. It's pretty difficult though I look in the mirror and see a mess. I'm not doing my job properly and I know it and I know others do too. One more week and it's half term. I think I'll get my hair cut and buy new clothes – sounds corny but perhaps it'll help.

Afraid the crazy one is me. I am not coping. My job is tough at present and I know I'm not as efficient as I was. My heart is at home and school comes second or third or further down the line. Life is hard between Mike and myself. Mike is under the same pressure as me and I can see his way of remaining sane is to carry on whatever. He needs to stick to routine and this provides security. I have tried to support this. However, I want some love and attention too. Perhaps I am not giving enough but I haven't any more strength. That's all I can write now as I'm a bit mixed up at the moment.

My week has been pathetic to begin with. Following my last pitiful cry at the top of the page I got worse and shouted at Betty [Auntie Betty] and Mike at the weekend. I felt so tense and could not cope or should I say did not want to cope with her. We have got to a point where Sunday is no longer a day off. I know it puts more of a burden on Mike and his dad but just now I don't want to know.

Well, that's all for now. This saga is turning into a story of self pity. I will overcome it.

Since last putting pen to paper I have been a complete idiot – a selfish stupid confused woman – moving to someone who was so insecure it was unbelievable – to a very caring wife and mother (which I hope I always was) – to someone who had sorted out her priorities – to today where I know where these priorities really are.

I've had a rough time – confused over Mike's attitude towards me in preference for his dad and Betty. It hurts –

My wonderful family are the most precious things on this earth. Each one backing up the other. I feel at times that I'm the weak link. I know Mike sees me as a burden – he even listed me as one of his problems – I've tried to be stronger since then . . . Mike said last week that Paul embarrassed [him] by his drinking! I was shocked. I have only pride for him whatever he does – he goes out and lives! That takes lots and lots of guts – especially tonight.

I love him so much and he's nearly better – today seemed to crack him up – Knowing he was so near yet so far. I must find lots more strength to keep him going and back Mike up too. Tonight I need to sleep – tomorrow will be a long hard day! Mike is restless – I must sort him out.

Sitting in a lovely house at South Erradale on holiday. The decision to come and leave Paul and the family far behind was long and painful. Mike desperately needed a break but I wanted to stay home. I know this holiday will build us up for the months ahead. Since I last wrote the emotions have been many.

Sadly today I write because I need to put my feelings on paper. I cannot understand what is going on. Mike is being unpleasant, no, unsympathetic towards Paul. I cannot really explain and do not know what to do.

Paul has said tonight that as soon as he is well enough, he's leaving!! I'm devastated. I know I've smothered him but Mike is the opposite and made him unwelcome. He says for the last two weeks Mike's made it clear to him that he's not welcome. I can't believe this. Only a few weeks ago Paul was near to death and suddenly, now he's alive he's not wanted!!!

What is he playing at!

I know we all need to adjust and it's been difficult with so many people visiting our little house to accommodate everyone, but surely it's worth the sacrifice. I don't know whether I'm right or wrong but I cannot accept Mike's attitude. When we were 23 we wanted to be free to live our lives as we wished. To be with friends, to go to bed late, to be noisy, etc, etc. Paul has no choice at present other than to depend on us, but he wants to begin to live life as a normal 23 year old. What is Mike up to? If Paul goes because of him – I shall not forgive him. From now I shall watch – I've let Mike know how I feel tonight and if there's no change I shall react as in the past. I only wish I was younger.

I wrote in the past about the difficulties families faced when illness came. I had failed to see the problems which could arise as things got better. I can see Mike's viewpoint a little, as he does not want _his_ life disturbed. What he fails to remember is how he has disturbed others in the past. Also Paul is trying to pick up the pieces of life whilst still being ill – he has a long, long way to go yet and still needs the security of our home to build on.

He has my blessing all the way.

I think from now on I need to consider not only Paul's future but my own. I think I'll help Paul find a flat or somewhere so's he can go to Poly if he wants. I couldn't bear him to leave W-ton yet I know he'll go eventually but I don't want him forced out by Mike – I want him to go when he's ready.

(Sue B)

There is much evidence here of Sue B feeling rejected and criticized by her husband. She speaks of him as 'My dear Mike' which suggests love and affection, and it is with pain and hurt that she relates his criticism of her. Sue B acknowledges that Mike's way of keeping sane is to stick to his routine. In George's story, his mother tells us that this was the way that George's father coped – by always having work to do. Whereas in George's family, though his parents coped in different ways, it was apparently without blame or rancour, clearly this was not the situation between Sue B and Mike. Again we can see echoes of the discussion in the first chapter, where different coping mechanisms are misunderstood by the other partner and serve to drive a wedge between them. There are many other nuances in this account, to which the reader will relate on a personal level, but it seems that, the overriding message is that the family is in crisis. The pain each feels is unbearable. The roller coaster of emotion, of hope and despair leave the members of the family unable to help themselves or each other.

Charlotte gives a further account of marital disharmony. Again we see blame and counter blame:

I also blame my husband who is very controlling and insisted he took Sean to the GP of his choice (his friend). He had told Sean he need not listen to his mother (me) if he did not wish. Sean told my husband, I found out later, not to let the doctor fob him off – it was serious. My husband believed the doctor who said, it was all right. (My husband is abusive and cruelly manipulative to me too). Later my husband encouraged Sean to sue the doctor(s), who he blamed. The doctor was at fault, negligent medically, but we were at fault, morally too. Had my husband and I been communicating, Sean may have told us more and sooner; I could have impressed our concern to the doctor more deeply – more than my husband did. I blame myself, but I blame my husband much more. It will always be between us although I do not say anything.

There came a point with Sean when investigations accelerated and then we were told it was cancer. I felt shock, guilt, that I had not acted on my instincts (although that was difficult with my awkward, controlling husband), but was very positive. By the acceleration of events I should have thought it was cancer (my husband did) but I had gone off this idea, thinking it was infection or something, like the doctors. My husband and I were abrasive to each other (he was worse) with the strain. I am suffering loss now.

> My husband appears to be coping. He probably off-loads to his school nurse as well as on me in round-about ways.
>
> This has added a strain to our relationship. Really, both I and my husband need help separately as well as together. I think we should part. What do I mean by 'help?' I do not really know, and I do not think anyone else does either. I suppose the answer is understanding.
>
> (Charlotte)

We see here a marriage in crisis: the word 'blame' is used repeatedly, Charlotte blames herself; she blames her husband; and they both blame the doctor. However, Charlotte refers to her husband as 'abusive, manipulative and controlling' and it is unlikely that these are traits that were manifested only after the advent of Sean's illness. Again the situation appears to suggest a relationship with problems which were thrown into sharp relief by the illness.

Rosenblatt (2000a) addresses the effect on the sexual aspects of a marital relationship after the death of a child, which, as we saw in the first chapter, can be far-reaching. In the following passage, which appears to refer to a loving and supportive partnership, Gabrielle refers to the impact on her sexuality:

> The only thing that still eludes me is my libido. I want sex but feel nothing. Poor Richard, he needs it so much so I go through the motions. I haven't deceived him. I am honest about how I feel. It is not mental. I love being held and touched and stroked and loved, I just don't feel sexual.
>
> (Gabrielle)

We have heard other mothers talk of emotional distance, and resentments between them and their partners, however, this is the first mention of the effect of death on sexuality and libido. It is not possible to tell if this is because it has not been an issue for other parents, or whether because it is such a sensitive and private subject that it has been avoided. We may assume that where relationships have broken down the cessation of a sexual relationship might well be part of that breakdown. However, Gabrielle's relationship with Richard appears in all other ways to be sound.

Lynn's relationship with her husband Ray has also been affected, though she says they have always been close.

> The very fabric of parenting has been destroyed, my role of parent to a son has been taken from me and I feel that a part of my own existence has been destroyed, nothing has meaning and I feel a deep despair . . . Ray and I have always been close but the pain of grief can sometimes drive a wedge between us. It is difficult to share our loss and support each other, we both have our own ways of grieving.

I need words whilst Ray needs silence and our tears are unbearably painful as we hurt so much it is difficult to hold each other's pain.

(Lynn)

There is much in this passage that echoes the way in which other contributors have expressed emotions. That Lynn's husband needs 'silence' whilst she needs 'words' relates to other narratives, to George's story and to the discussion in Chapter 1 about the gendered response to grief. Whilst it might seem that the one person who could truly understand the pain, the loss and the grief, would be the other parent, as Lynn points out, they both hurt so much they have no resources to support each other. However, another account speaks of the strengthening of family bonds:

Quite apart from recognition that the whole family have gone through abnormal situations and I would submit become the better and closer for these experiences. Throughout it all we had a lot of laughs along the way. Parents probably play the most important unsung role of being supportive to one another.

(Donald and Annie)

Donald and Annie had to cope with a cancer diagnosis with both of their daughters, both thankfully survived, and it seems that what was already a strong family was further strengthened by their ordeal. Again this suggests that pre-existing relationships have a fundamental impact on the effect of the illness.

Reflections

This chapter, unlike those that precede it, has not been based on the life stage of the young adult with cancer; rather it has focused on the parental relationships and the impact of the illness on them. However, although many of the issues addressed here might apply equally to parents facing the life-threatening illness or death of a child at any age, when added to the particular problems created by life-stage factors the impact on the marriage may be more far-reaching. If parents already have to manage the disruption to family dynamics, which have been so powerfully expressed through the narratives in this book so far, any fragility in their relationship is likely to be exacerbated.

In the narrative material there is evidence of blame, self-blame and mutual recrimination between partners. Only one narrative speaks of the family becoming stronger, whilst several tell us of marriages that have failed, or have been put under immense strain. Again, Rosenblatt's (2000a, 2000b) work in this area suggests that such effects are to be expected (see Chapter 1).

Only one narrative addressed the resumption of a sexual relationship after the death, but this may have been an issue for other couples too. Rosenblatt (2000a) says that after the death of a child many couples experience a break in their sexual relationship. Low energy levels, emotional distance, depression and resistance to pleasure all contribute to a loss of libido. According to Rosenblatt, some couples resume sexual intercourse as a result of it being the woman's primary goal to conceive. Although no parents whose stories are told in this book have supplied their ages, it is probable, given the age of their lost children, that many parents are in their 40s or 50s. This suggests that a significant proportion will be at an age and life stage where further procreation is less likely to be an option.

However, not all the accounts tell us of the failure of a marriage, and those stories which do relate experiences of hostility and marital disruption also tend to suggest that there were pre-existing problems. Where a marriage has been 'hanging on by a thread' or where there have been significant resentments or differences that predate the illness, it is clear that the illness has not succeeded in bringing the couple closer together. Indeed this would be unlikely; as even in those marriages that have survived there is an acknowledgement that each partner has been so damaged by the experience that they are the one with least resources to offer the other. Again this reflects Rosenblatt's work. However, where the partnership has been strong, despite differences in coping strategies – commonly the man being unable or unwilling to articulate his feelings whilst the woman wants to talk about her fears and emotions – the upheaval has not threatened the relationship. In such cases each partner has allowed the other the space to adopt a particular role in relationship to the illness and its management without necessarily articulating the difference to the other.

Gender is clearly a central issue in this chapter, as Walter (1996) argues, there is evidence that men and women grieve in different ways, though most theories of grief are based on grieving women. This may precipitate problems as Brabant, Forsythe and McFarlain (1994) say that where parents have contradictory perceptions of the nature of the family following a child's death they experience greater problems. Riches and Dawson (2000) observe that the majority of research studies suggest that fathers are more likely after bereavement to put their energies into practical tasks whilst mothers are more likely to connect with their feelings and to express strong emotion. Though these authors also caution us that generalizations can be dangerous, such a position would appear to be supported by the narratives in this chapter and can be seen to cause problems between parents. The research of Reay, Bignold, Ball and Cribb (1998) suggests that the adoption of gender roles represents an 'exaggerated normality' and that such gender patterns raise difficult issues within heterosexual relationships. The result is 'emotional distance, incomprehension and interpersonal friction' (1998: 51).

So, what can be done to support partners undergoing such a crisis? Riches and Dawson suggest that we are poorly equipped as a society to deal with loss, and that the intellectual models available ill-prepare us to know how it feels to lose a child. They argue that those who work with bereaved families need to be able to contemplate their own deaths and – even more difficult – the deaths of our children. They also provide a summary of support principles that include the following:

- Attention should be directed not only at the individuals but also the relationship contexts
- Talking is a key resource for making sense of death
- Differences in grieving need to be appreciated
- Fathers tend to be overlooked
- Grief can produce resentments that exacerbate pre-existing problems
- The acceptability of 'time off' from grief should be confirmed
- Supporters should not forget the positive outcome of sharing the challenge of the death.

(Riches and Dawson 2000: 74–5)

Marital relationships may be less likely to be discussed with health professionals than the other effects of the illness that are addressed in this book. However, if health professionals are aware of the likely effects on a marriage, they may be able to suggest counselling, if appropriate, or at least offer reassurance that tensions are to be expected under the circumstances. As Rosenblatt (2000a: 111) says, 'Finding out what is "normal" can be reassuring as you learn that others have had to deal with the same pain and frustration.'

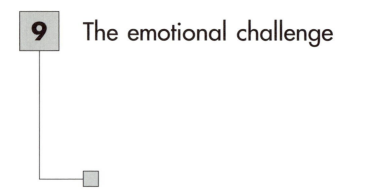

9 The emotional challenge

George's story

Well I think, really for me there were two distinct situations, one was the emotional impact of George's illness and dying which I have to separate out from the emotional impact of bereavement. So first of all when I remember the emotional impact of the four years of his illness it was a most physical experience. I can't really remember the anxiety, the uncertainty and the despair without remembering all the physical symptoms of insomnia, of disrupted digestion, of shallow breathing, of palpitations, of sweating, of having a huge lump in my chest all the time, that was how it affected me – at a very, very physical level. The relief I got from those feelings was really only achieved by doing things for George. And of course often the last thing George wanted was for me to do things for him. He wanted to be independent and separate. I mean . . . he knew that as well as carrying my own pain at the possibility of losing him or indeed at what he had to face in terms of treatment, he knew I was also carrying the pain that he felt and this was very hard for him but there was no way I could avoid it. It was like the sort of situation when he was little and he got missed out of the playground games or didn't get invited to go to the sleep-over, it was the same sort of feeling but a million times worse. But here he was, as a young man, facing horrendous treatments and surgery and the possibility of death. So it was hard. And after he died I only had to cope with my own pain, which in many ways has been much easier.

So when I reflect back I remember the physical symptoms but I also remember the pain that George himself went through, especially his emotional pain and I remember the dates on the calendar for the reviews which were always three monthly and how hard those were for him and how on a number of occasions he got the bad news that he was dreading.

There was a definite change for me about three years after diagnosis. George got a recurrence of lung secondaries really quite large and aggressive lung secondaries. And that occurred in March '98 and he died in March '99. And as soon as those metastases were found on the X-rays I 'knew' that he couldn't survive, so all of the uncertainty of the previous three years, the hope and the fear and the check-ups, the possibility of a future and the possibility of death all suddenly evaporated. And for the last 12 months of his life I knew that in a sense what was important was the quality of that end part of George's life. How we as a family and he as an individual used the time and how he himself coped with increasing disability and debility. And it seems strange to say, but it was actually easier for me because I knew then what we had to do and all the uncertainty had gone. I think, I felt quite isolated at that time though, because until the last six months of his life Geoff and Jonathan and most of the people close to us still seemed to be of the belief that George could be cured. But I felt certain that he couldn't. So it wasn't really until the last few months that Geoff came to the same understanding that I had reached. George himself still believed that he could live until about 10 days before he died and that was fine. During that time what was important to me was the quality of George's life and the fact that by the end of it he would have found peace of mind and acceptance and equanimity and that was what in fact he did. And having worried for four years and known for 12 months that he would die the fact that he died at home and peacefully was for me I suppose a huge achievement for George himself and a huge family achievement. So at the point of bereavement there was enormous relief. I now feel myself to be in a category of bereaved people who've lost someone they love. But while he was ill I felt myself to be in a very special and unusual and unique category of people who were actually watching a child going through the most challenging of physical and emotional experiences and that felt very different. Now that I'm a bereaved parent I suppose I have made mental adjustments that allow me to still see ourselves as a family with three sons, one of whom has died. We find ways of including George in as many of our family occasions and I suppose in our daily lives as possible. The research project and book have been invaluable in allowing me to take the experience of George's illness into a future. As a family we are able to talk about him, to say, 'that was George's T-shirt or George liked that chocolate cake or do you remember when we went to such and such a place?' We don't have a problem, we call his bedroom 'George's room' we are able to talk about him relatively freely and we always find ways of referring to him on special occasions. Things that I suppose I hadn't anticipated was that I would become very physically ill after he died.

Although I did know during the last few weeks of caring for him at home that I was becoming increasingly unwell and at one point I felt so ill that I thought I was going to die before him. And in fact that was something that I knew I couldn't allow to happen but after he died it didn't matter to me terribly much. I feel better now physically. Looking at how I feel now I suppose the changes are that I have absolutely no fear of dying at all, none whatsoever. I tend to be able to live one day at a time without planning very far ahead, which is something that I didn't do before. I don't listen to music, I don't go to the theatre unless I know what the play's going to be about and that I will be able to cope with it. I don't read fiction, I don't watch fiction on television because I think that I am probably at the limit of what I can cope with emotionally and therefore have an anxiety of being tipped over into emotional over-load by the vicarious experiences of other people through novels, films, plays. So these are things that I avoid. I imagine this will improve with time but they are things that I used to enjoy, certainly before George got ill. I try to avoid going to places that were special to George, especially places that were special during his illness because I find that too hard. I can't imagine ever going back to Zennor in Cornwall or to Arnside, near home, where we used to drive out so he could look across Morecambe Bay. These were things that we did in the last few months of George's life and it would be too painful to do them again. But somehow – I don't know – I just accept that that's the way that life will now be and I don't worry that it should or could have been different, this is just the way it is.

This chapter has a different format than the preceding chapters that have been organized around individual themes. There is no single theme here. Rather it presents material from the narratives which expresses the emotional impact of life-threatening illness in a young adult child, and addresses the problems associated with finding ways of coping with the tragedy of illness and loss.

Many of the quotations used are lengthy. This is necessary to allow the depth and range of feeling to be communicated. There is an attempt to group the extracts around the various issues raised, but as many of the narratives address overlapping themes, this cannot be the basis on which the material is organized. The narratives are so powerful that additional commentary is kept to a minimum.

Friends don't understand

The thread that runs through the first narrative extracts is one which reflects on the impossibility of others understanding the pain, grief and loss experienced by parents who have lost a young adult child to cancer. We begin with an extract from Moira's narrative, about the death of her son Alasdair at the age of 19, whilst he was a student. Where she used capital letters and underlining in her original text these have been reproduced to show the strength of feeling and emotion behind the words.

Our friends have been wonderful, but Bill and I can't come to terms with the fact that Alasdair was snatched away just as he was beginning to achieve, to live. No-one understands this. They can't. A friend who lost her husband when he was 52 tries to compare this – Jim had a lot of life left to live. BUT HE <u>HAD</u> A LIFE – ALASDAIR DIDN'T GET A CHANCE. She <u>doesn't</u> understand she didn't watch her child suffer agony and be helpless to do anything about it.

We badly need to be in touch with someone who knows the HELL we are going through even 6½ months down the line. I don't seem to be getting over him at all. I still cry every night. I still want to scream and shout and kick – which so far I have <u>not</u> done. I just <u>want</u> to.

The hospice are wonderful. But this is new territory for them. He was the youngest patient they ever had. Which is why so many of the staff were upset and attended the funeral – something they never do apparently. But at least we know Alasdair died loved and surrounded by love in the hospice. You could almost touch the love . . . I am trying to tell myself that I had a bonus having Alasdair for 19 years since really only a big meal at my gran's on 23rd September 1979 stopped Monblands Hospital in Airdrie taking me to theatre after I'd had a dreadful haemorrhage at my gran's house. They left me till morning, when the consultant found that the cervix was closed, therefore I was probably still pregnant.

(Moira)

It is clear from Moira's account that despite well-meaning attempts at offering sympathy, friends – whom it is acknowledged have been 'wonderful' – cannot understand her pain and loss. In fact the more friends try to empathize, the more Moira feels they cannot comprehend the extent of her anguish, thus she feels the need for support from those who understand what they have suffered and continue to suffer. Similarly in the passage from Elizabeth below she comments that unless a person has been through the loss of a child they cannot comprehend the pain:

I know now I couldn't go through that again not on my own. What hurt me most is that I couldn't do nothing at all for Michael only be at his side 24 hours a day. What I am trying to say is when you got a child who is very poorly you haven't got a life for yourself. I will never forget what Michael and I have been through for those 3½ years, it is like going to hell and back, not knowing what's going to happen next. People make me laugh, they say they know what we have been through but they don't. If they haven't had a child with cancer they don't know nothing. I just wish one day someone from the government would go to Leeds Hospital and go on the ward to see all the sick children and the parents, see how they would feel seeing young children and parents not knowing if their child is going to live or die . . . This is from my heart. I loved Michael very much but I still cannot come to terms with this, that Michael had died. It is five months now and I still cry for him. I just wish I could have done more for him then he might have still been here today with his brother John and myself.

I just wish Michael will R.I.P.
Love always from my heart.
I will always love you Michael you were very brave.
And I am proud of you and I know all your friends think so as well.

I know that Michael will be missed but he is still in my heart. When I go to his grave I always talk to him, asking him things and telling him how much I love him and miss him.

(Elizabeth)

Although narratives in the previous chapter indicate that having a partner is not necessarily the support it 'should' be, clearly being a single parent brings its own problems as we see from Elizabeth's account; and at some level she appears to feel that had she been able to do 'more' for him he might still be alive. This is clearly not the case, but as a mother, responsible for her child's well-being since his birth, it is an understandable response to feel that she should have been able to protect him.

Carol, herself a trained counsellor, could not tolerate the prospect of counselling with a person who could only imagine her grief. Yet again we see that the well-meaning offers of sympathy and support from those who *think* they can empathize are intolerable:

What could have helped at the time? After Sara died, my doctor offered counselling. I refused it – I was a trained counsellor myself: somehow I couldn't face words of sympathy from someone who could only <u>imagine</u> how it felt and not <u>know</u>. Anyhow, I have a belief that what we need are less therapists and more therapeutic people! But would it have helped? Perhaps. During Sara's illness, I hadn't requested a Macmillan nurse. This puzzles me now since we had had one when my mother was living with cancer – over seven years, many of them with us. I know she had found her nurse, Sue, a great comfort and support so why hadn't I asked for another 'Sue?' Perhaps I had mistakenly tried to be everything for Sara – perhaps too, I had denied the notion that she might die: it was too awful to contemplate. Whatever the reason, I regret it now. I remember meeting a mother in the hospital whose son (he was 18) had been receiving treatment for osteosarcoma. 'How old is your daughter?' she asked. When I told her, she replied 'The outcome for David isn't too promising; he's doing well now, but...At least you've had your daughter for 25 years'. I don't know if David survived his cancer or not. Perhaps we should have stayed in touch. I would not have welcomed a parents' support group whilst Sara was ill, but I think it did help to meet another mother in a similar position. I didn't feel so isolated, so unusual, so alone. It was happening in other families too. Maybe there should be organisations offering to put parents in touch with each other locally, details being displayed in hospitals, Oncology clinics? I 'phoned the Lymphoma Helpline once. The nurse was sympathetic but clearly not able to give me hope. One morning when I felt impossibly low, I contacted my local Samaritans branch. 'My dear, I just want to give you a hug', the volunteer said. I've always remembered her words.

(Carol)

In a letter to Helen, Denise C also acknowledges the fact that no one who has not lost a child can understand her pain:

It was a great consolation to hear that you can identify with my feelings about Alexander's courage and my pride in him causing me to get so upset. No-one else seemed to understand this or at least not be able to put their feelings into words.

(Denise C)

We have seen that friends' well-meaning attempts to offer comfort can be insensitive, and parents may feel an instinctive need to seek contact with others who have experienced a similar loss. However, there is a tension here between this need and Carol's acknowledgement that she would not have wanted to be in touch with a parents' support group during the illness. This may reflect a need for a semblance of 'normality'. Denise articulates this dichotomy:

Sometimes I did feel I did not want to be with others in similar situations. I wanted to just be a normal, healthy family...Laura was a pupil at the local High School in Ashington and unfortunately and unbelievably there have been other children affected with cancer and so we do have close contact with at least one other family – this can be a great comfort – as only they can relate to and know how you really feel.

(Denise)

This passage reflects the confusion and possibly changing needs of parents. At some stages they probably do need to be with others who have experienced the same grief, and at those times, well-meaning friends who do not share those experiences are a source of irritation. Yet we also see that Denise recognizes at other times the importance of 'normality' and does not want to be 'ghettoized'. Chapter 3 established the importance of normality for the young adults and to some extent the parents too. Here it is articulated in a way that indicates how difficult it is to identify what might be of help. Not only will different families require different kinds of support, that support may vary during the course of the bereavement process.

The need for continued contact with the hospice movement

The belief that only those who have experienced a similar loss can truly understand may lead bereaved parents to seek continued contact with the hospice where their son or daughter was treated, sometimes as a volunteer, or to undertake other cancer-related charity work:

> To cut a long and rather harrowing period short I have subsequently remarried and now work as a Bereavement Co-ordinator/Counsellor for Cancer Care. (I had always been involved with working with young people, parents, etc in all sorts of guises – youth work, sex education, drugs – and this seemed a natural step). It hasn't, isn't always easy but I feel that losing a child can either destroy you <u>or</u> you have to find something from it which ultimately you can use to help others . . . Even now, more than five years on, I berate myself for things I can't now alter. Why did we glibly explain away her early tiredness because Sara's job involved working shifts? Why was her back pain 'diagnosed' as a trapped nerve? It had been a warning of something more sinister and we'd all ignored it. I remember driving her home from the hospital when the cancer had finally reached her lungs – her lungs for God's sake, why not anywhere but her lungs? Sara asked in a quiet voice, 'Mum am I going to die?' I replied 'No, you're <u>not</u>' in a voice that tried to convince us both, but deep down I think we both knew. That night, I slept in Sara's bed, aware that if I held her too close I might (again) dislodge her Hickman line. 'What shall we do, Sara?' I asked. 'Just give me a hug,' she said. 'What about the Hickman?' 'Oh damn the Hickman'. She died six weeks later.
>
> (Carol)

It appears that in this case using the experience to help others has helped Carol to carry on. This is true of a number of instances where continued work with the hospice movement has acted as a support to bereaved parents. Candy, who lost both her husband and her daughter within a short period, reflects on the stress and peoples' response to her plight. She too has found continued contact and volunteer work with the hospice to be an emotional support:

When my husband died friends tried to keep me going by reassuring me that life would get better and then Sianne got cancer and they really became lost, there was no more they could say and everyone virtually backed away because THEY COULDN'T COPE! No-one even offered to do any washing, etc. for me. I think the enormity of the situation made them forget that on top of everything else I still had a family to look after and a house to run! . . . I think perhaps one thing that helped me cope was the fact that I rarely had time to think about anything it was just one crisis after another. I didn't have the luxury of time on my hands to worry. I have to say that without the amazing support of the Family Support Group at my local hospice I wouldn't have stayed sane, if that's the right term! On top of all this we were moving. We had wanted to move since my husband died and as fate decreed everything was moving during Sianne's last weeks. We actually moved just over two weeks after Sianne died. At least I knew that Sianne really wanted the move too and that even if only briefly she had visited our new home. Lots of people were very negative about the move telling me I couldn't handle the added stress. However, one of my supports at the hospice told me that I really couldn't be under anymore stress than with Sianne in the hospice and she gave me the confidence to go through with it. I don't regret the move but at the moment feel so desolate that I don't think it would make much difference where I lived . . . There is such a terrible feeling of inadequacy and failure because the one thing you should be able to do is to protect your child but cancer robs you of this gift. I found losing my child was so infinitely more devastating than losing my husband but at the time of his death I believed that I had experienced the worst life could throw at me. I still find it so hard to come to terms with why it had to be Sianne when the disease was so rare and I had already lost her dad. She had so much potential and personality. She was loved by so many, she was popular, artistic and doing well at college . . . I am still in contact with the St Helena Hospice as a volunteer and also for support for me and my children when we need it. Sometimes it helps me through just to know that there is someone I can talk to, who understands what I am trying to struggle through.

(Candy)

We see here, that Candy's friends appear to have been overwhelmed by the tragedies in her life and rendered incapable of supporting her.

What seems to have given her strength is her continued contact with the hospice where Sianne died, where people understand her struggle and pain. Although in this case not as a volunteer, continuing attachment to the hospice where Simon died is also reflected on by Helen V:

> The chaplain of the hospice took the funeral with the help of the local Anglican vicar who we'd asked for. We had no particular wish for a special funeral, since it was so far from home and we were still struggling with shock. Yet it became special. We were urged to use the hospice chapel, a small, beautiful centuries-old domed building with a side entrance off the corridor near Simon's room. Nurses came. I'd asked that they not bring flowers; I felt they'd done everything to care for him, and that was enough. But Nicola and Debbie brought roses, an apricot-coloured bunch with a hand-written note: 'A short time in our lives, forever in our hearts'. Tyson and Peter gave us a gift too, in joining the procession into the chapel behind Simon's coffin . . . The crematorium was a dismal experience. There were vast arrays of flowers, all fake except for those on Simon's coffin. There was even a quavery electronic organ. It was so hard to let Simon go. I'd said I didn't want the coffin to slide back out of sight, so we just sat through the brief ceremony, copied the priest in sprinkling holy water on the coffin, and then left.
>
> Afterwards, we went to lunch with Peter and Tyson, at the Italian restaurant where they'd been with my brother only a week before. Patrick and I had been hoping they would tell us all about Simon's last days, but Patrick pressed them too hard and it was the wrong time. The only thing they said was that Simon had thought about making a will in the last week, and wanted Peter to have his treasured computer game set-up.
>
> We, or at least, I will always want to know what it was like for Simon in those days in London. Patrick feels he must have woken every morning to the thought that death was near. I just don't know, but I have an enormous respect for the care he was given at the hospice. The nurses were loving, the doctor compassionate and caring. The receptionist/administrator, Sandra, was endlessly helpful and understanding – quite special. They allowed Simon to face the end courageously. I feel he was able to keep on joking with his friends almost to the last because he could tell the staff his fears (reading between the lines of his file).
>
> Perhaps I'm too attached to the hospice. But they continue to help me to grieve, and I feel I still need them. Paula sent us a water-colour from London that reminded her of Simon. The chance to write this story came through the social worker at the hospice. The memory of Simon seems to live on there.

The staff and Tyson and Peter did what I would have liked to do – they accompanied Simon through his dying. Simon was wise in going to London. These people weren't his parents, they loved him and cared for him as if they were.

(Helen V)

We remember that Simon died in London soon after his diagnosis in Australia, and his mother did not see him alive again after his departure with his friends. Here she draws comfort from contact with the people who cared for him, as she would have liked to do, yet she manages to say that 'Simon was wise in going to London'. At least she knows that he spent his last weeks living life to the full, seeing sights that he would not have had the chance to see had he stayed with his family, and Helen V draws some comfort from this too.

We have already seen that continued involvement in the hospice movement through voluntary work has given a purpose to parents after their son or daughter's death. Below is an account of charitable work somewhat outside the hospice environment undertaken by parents, which has given them a focus of activity, and kept them in contact with others who have a real understanding of their loss.

On 31st May 1997, Mat died. He had developed pneumonia. His suffering was horrendous. But he left us with so many happy memories. He was our hero. We were privileged to have known him and to have shared his life.

This young man touched the hearts of so many people. It was his wish that we raise money to help others with bone cancer. This is why Matthew's Beacon has been established.

Because bone cancer is so rare; because it affects only a few people; funds are not so readily available so Matthew's Beacon is hoping to raise funds to help research a cure or improve the treatment for bone cancer. This was Matthew's wish – he asked us to do this for him – it was one of the promises he asked us to make . . .

No one should dismiss cancer of any kind, thinking it will never happen to me. It happened to our family. It continues to strike at other innocent victims. By raising money, we can hope to advance a cure, and perhaps more people will survive. Perhaps Matthew will not have died for nothing.

(Iris)

It is apparent that Matthew's Beacon is both a memorial to her lost son, and a way in which Iris hopes others might be helped. It helps to bring something positive from tragedy, as Iris says 'perhaps Matthew will not have died for nothing'.

The trivial nature of everyday life

The need to remain in contact with those who have shared the experience through voluntary work in a hospice or through contact with other parents in a support group, may be one way of coping with the essentially 'trivial' nature of everyday life. The quotation from Barbara below is prefaced earlier in her narrative by the phrase 'At that time I was a married woman' suggesting that her marriage did not survive the period when her son was ill, though in fact her son did survive. What we see from this extract is the irritation that is felt at the importance attributed to 'unimportant' events:

> I would sit watching the 'Good Morning' programme with Richard and Judy and hell what did it matter what was the fashion that Christmas? Who cared whether she had a bag to match her dress? Who the hell gives a damn as to what to buy your best friend for Christmas, do I care about the price of brussel sprouts, for God's sake don't you all know, can't you all see that I am suffering here, I am dying quietly inside. My son is dying . . . what's wrong with this world? You have no right to be happy . . . I am not happy, my family are not happy . . . and so it continued.
>
> And then the Lockerbie disaster occurred. Like millions of others I sat watching on TV the dreadful scenes of the carnage, the desperation, the sadness and total loss . . . and then quite suddenly I began to cry . . . and I cried non-stop for a week. And to this day I don't know why it happened the way it did . . . Hell, you don't ever expect your children to die before you . . .
>
> I often think back to those dark days, but you try not to dwell in the past too much. You are all too grateful for the love and comfort that family and friends offered then, and have nothing but admiration for the medical and nursing staff who cared so lovingly for your child . . . Sometimes I believe that whilst I have no answer as to why these things happen, I believe that when they do it is up to each of us to delve deep down inside ourselves to try and find the strength and courage that we are going to need. And I believe that if we are fortunate to be able to draw from that courage and strength, then hopefully, we become stronger and better within ourselves . . . but it's a hard price to pay.
>
> (Barbara)

Here it is apparent that the trivia of everyday life is an affront. Things which assume importance to others, such as what to wear, what to eat, planning for Christmas enrage parents who are facing the death of their child. However, unlike some of the other accounts where the parents have felt strongly that the comfort offered by friends was misguided and meaningless, Barbara tells us how grateful she was for such support while acknowledging that the strength to continue has to be dredged up from somewhere deep inside.

Lynn documents a similar response to the trivia of everyday life. This passage begins with an account of the devastation caused by Simon R's illness:

> It all seemed straightforward so why was I feeling like shite? Those early days travelling backwards and forwards to Southampton were so very traumatic I fail to recall how I got through it. The seriousness of the situation we all found ourselves in was so frightful I almost hoped we would be wiped out on the M3 by some wanker in a BMW – at least I would not have the wild thoughts and macabre images already mapped out in my mind as Simon's existence for the next 12 weeks.
>
> How do I tell my family, how do I tell my friends, what do I say to my employer, how about acquaintances or those cretins who pester you with telephone sales.
>
> *'Good afternoon Mrs Robinson, my name is Tracey and I am phoning on behalf of ABC continental apartments. This is your lucky day – you have been chosen to partake in a free holiday in one of our luxury apartments in the Costa Del Sol . . .' Stop right there bitch! This is certainly not my lucky day as my son has been diagnosed with cancer, his prolonged treatment prevents me from taking any sort of holiday away from the hospital and should you phone again with such mind-numbing trivia I shall make it my duty to shove this phone up your arse – now piss off and leave me alone! – Or words to that effect anyway.*
>
> Being the coward I am I left it to Manda to break the bad news to all and sundry as I am still fighting with the belief that it is all my fault as I must have done/not done something during his short life to cause this nightmare. Apparently, cancer is foetal and is formed in the foetus during conception. As the sperm touches the ovum, rogue cells are made and lay in wait to pounce later in life. Little bastards. Maybe it was because I smoked around him but whatever the statistics or medical theories or hocus-pocus cause, I know that in some way I must have contributed to the nightmare . . . why Simon? I have tortured my mind whilst searching for reasons why, he does not deserve this.
>
> (Lynn)

This extract raises many issues that the reader will relate to on a personal level, and Lynn's re-enactment of an imaginary phone call from a telesales person yet again demonstrates, with an acerbic wit, the irritation caused by such trivia. It is also clear that there is a need to find a 'reason' for the loss, and a tendency to attribute blame for the inexplicable. In this case Lynn blames herself in an attempt to make sense of the nonsensical.

The following passage tells of us of how Lynn and her family have attempted to come to terms with Simon R's death:

When Simon died another journey to hell took place just as it did when we first heard about the diagnosis. A phase of life came to an end and Simon's illness, which had been the focus for 20 months of our lives suddenly no longer had any significance. We are left with a great void. We had to plan the funeral, inform family, friends, and officials that Simon had died and the intense concern of keeping Simon alive was wiped out and it is so difficult to come to terms with reality and adjusting to the loss of structure and purpose to each day. It is difficult to re-enter the world of every day practicalities which seem to dominate 'normal' families and which now seem so trivial in the face of our tragic loss of Simon. But we are still here, still attempting to carry on with life as 'normal'. We have lovely memories of Simon to reflect on when we feel desperate and thankfully, audio and video tapes to lean on when times get really hard. It is very complex to grieve as a family. We hold so much collective pain, the amputation is unbearable for each one of us and yet it is also different because Simon was a son, brother, uncle, boyfriend, best mate, meaning something different to each one of us.

SO DARKENED AM I,

THAT ALL DAY MY DAY IS NIGHT

I count the days, weeks and months since he left us – it is 6 months now and still I think what now? Go back to work? Impossible. Carry on? Impossible. My only son is dead, never to see him again, never to hear 'Hi Stress' or 'Fat Boy'. I even miss 'Waaaaarrpppp'. Tears – how many? How often? For how long? How come the simple tasks are now impossible? The house is so quiet, how can I go to bed without saying goodnight to him? How do I wake up each day and face another day of agony? Why do I cry because there is no washing in the laundry basket? Why can't I do my shopping because I can't buy my usual things? Why can't I go out in the car without wanting to ram into a wall? Why is it so painful attending Saints matches? Why don't I play music anymore? I'm frightened I will hear 'those songs'. Why am I angry when people say 'Isn't it a beautiful day?'

It will never be beautiful again. What am I going to do with my aching arms? Why don't I feel normal? I want to feel normal – I never will again.

(Lynn)

Again the trivia of 'normal' life is commented on, yet paradoxically normality appears to be a goal. However in the final sentence Lynn says that, whilst she wants to feel normal, she believes that she never will again.

The enduring nature of the loss and pain

It may well be the case that Lynn's life will never be the same again as Mary whose daughter Nicola died some 20 years ago reflects on the lasting nature of the grief:

> I knew at the time she was ill that after she died would be the hardest part, that it would take for ever to reach any sort of peace after she'd gone. But that was for later not for now. Of course, you're never prepared for a death. And although I knew that the hardest part would come after she died, even so, I had no idea the pain would be so excruciating in the event. You're interested in how parents cope during the illness. I don't know. These days, I expect there's more communication. I couldn't talk to her or tell her how she had always been my life, my window on the world, talk about what a wonderful child she had been, for fear of touching the raw nerve underneath; I didn't want her to hear my voice falter or see my tears. I still can't talk about her, or write about her, without brimming eyes and falling tears. I think really that parents need someone to talk to, to weep to. That would probably be the healthiest thing for them, especially if they are the 'bottling up' type of person, as I am. I think there is no doubt that the young person is the brave one, the one who doesn't want to see her/his parents suffer, so tries to save them from that by being cheerful and accepting. At the end of the day, the young person's true colours come out, their sense of humour and their caring for others, especially their parents.
>
> (Mary)

Even after 20 years the pain is still fresh. There may be an expectation that time will lessen the pain of the loss. However, it can never be 'all right' to have lost a child, and although the grief finds a place, and parents continue with their lives and activities with an outward appearance of 'normality', the pain, as we see in Mary's' account, will never disappear entirely. The following extract from Joyce also suggests that the pain never goes away:

> They say time heals, but our story happened fourteen years ago on the 27th June 1986. I do not feel any different now that I did at the time. Grief is seasonal, with birthdays, anniversaries, Christmas and New Year. On every occasion there is always one missing, not just for us but all the family. The pain of losing Jill never goes away. We have had a lot of traumas in our lifetime, but living with cancer was definitely the worst. We are still emotional. I have found writing this, re-living it all in the words, not just thoughts, very draining.
>
> (Joyce)

For other readers whose bereavement is more recent, this passage and Mary's may seem profoundly depressing, as it is clear that the pain has not faded with the years for these respondents. For this reason I considered omitting such extracts. However, what Joyce and Mary say will resonate with many readers and some comfort may be drawn from their reaction. When such a loss has been experienced, perhaps there is too great a belief in an ability to 'move on'. The acuteness of emotions may change, but they will always be there, just below the surface, as Joyce says on birthdays or at Christmas, there will always be someone missing.

The following extract documents the struggles faced by Charlotte after Sean's death, a much more recent bereavement than those considered above:

It is nearly four months. There is a void. I think reaction is setting in but comes and goes. A girl who was in his group has sent an Easter card. I am loosely in touch with her and the group leader (aged thirty four). Both are still very shocked. Donna says she just cannot sing with anyone else drumming because it is not Sean. She is intending to arrange a charity concert for the hospital because of Sean. She may have me in it – I can sing folk. She also visits Sean's grave and talks to him – it is in easy reach for her. This may sound awful, but I have not visited Sean's grave yet. It is an awkward journey for me, but I do pray for him. My spiritual beliefs help.

Hilary and Chris continue to be supportive, and I need them. I have waves of sadness. A friend on the ward lost her daughter a few weeks later.

Ever since Sean died, I have been putting on a brave face. I am affected. I do as little work as possible around the house. My other children accept my explanation about Sean going. The school is very good to Ian who appears to cope well. I have been getting real abdominal pains but I think they are stress-related. I cannot read a novel or follow a plot on TV but I can read a textbook and follow documentaries. I have tried to distance myself with a part-time course. The course has helped the bereavement, but the bereavement has not helped the course. The tutors have been very understanding, so I think I am beginning to succeed in the course (after two failed assessments, I passed the third).

I have not had bereavement counselling yet, but I probably will. I am more often than not tired. I am not the same person as I was. I do not mean that negatively. A good friend of mine, a mother of three, came round yesterday and we casually started talking about God and death. I pointed out I hoped my spiritual beliefs are true (and not just beliefs) and that I was not frightened of death. She said 'spiritual beliefs' are true but she would be frightened of death. (I am middle aged and have enthusiasm to live). I said I saw things differently to her because I had lost a child. I do feel part of me has died, but this is probably shock. I am trying to resume interests. I am going to sing for at least two charities, solo, definitely. There is an awful lot to sing, so I am very excited. I have been asked to help distance learning (voluntarily) and that is very good for me.

Sean's illness and going have 'burnt me out' and I am not up to visiting my handicapped brother who now has no visitors. It is a shame, but I have written friendly letters and will visit when I can.

I socialize at a local cancer group. One day I would like to help bereaved people. There are many, many people in my position, probably worse.

Sean's needs and welfare were more important than my loss. He grew from a child to a man, then I lost him. My friend who lost her daughter, said her other one said 'H . . . and Sean would be chattering away happily together and with others where they are now, and looking at us'. I believe this too. Sean and young friends used not to 'believe in organised religion' as they put it, but confronted with mortality, spirituality became important. He was a beautiful person. Everyone loved him. I have lost a good friend too. It was a pleasure to care for him.

(Charlotte)

Charlotte's narrative displays many signs of grief as she tells us of the struggles she has had in managing life after Sean's death. However, as with other respondents in this chapter she too is undertaking voluntary work that she says is 'good for her' and it is clear that her spiritual beliefs have given her strength and support. We shall be returning to the issue of spirituality later in this chapter, but it seems that despite the anguish apparent in this extract, Charlotte's belief in God and the help the she has derived through religion seem to have been fundamental to her ability to cope with Sean's death.

One of the ways in which Gabrielle coped with the aftermath of Steve's death was to write to him, as though speaking directly to him. It is from these writings that all her contributions to this book have come:

I need to save all these personal things of yours. To save all the lovely cards and letters. So many people have written so many beautiful things about you, so full of fun and caring. The photos have been magic, showing a side of you I had never seen. All that larking about, the brilliant eye contact you had with people. You could make people feel very special, that's why you could sell. So many of your friends have written and given me photos, they loved you too . . . I loved your hands, Steve. You had long fingers and they were always so relaxed, this photo shows them beautifully . . . You all golden, all relaxed. The same smile, the same look, straight into the camera. You were very photogenic, Steve, aren't I lucky to have so many records of you. You were a real poser too!! Suddenly, today I was able to go and look at the two videos . . . How lovely it was to see you move again. See you run, laugh, joke and pose at the football charity match in August '97. Having fun at [a] 30th birthday party, drinking, playing games, chatting, relaxing and talking, just being you – alive.

It isn't easy, Steve. You asked 'What are you going to do when I'm gone, mum?' 'Just get on again', I said. But I can't get you out of my head. I expect to see you again. I look for you even though I know you have gone. I hear your voice greeting me as you come up the garden, 'Hi mum'. I see you kneeling by the pond watching the fish. I hear you whistling. I see you leaning against the work-surface in the kitchen drinking a beer. Your washing in a heap on the floor. Help me Steve! You were so strong. I know I owe it to you to be strong too. I owe it to Richard . . . and myself too. It is just so hard without you around. You consumed my life at the end. I couldn't clean, cook, iron, garden, exercise, work or read the paper. I kept myself looking OK or you would have noticed and commented. Now I have to get all these things back. Now I have to reclaim myself. It is just so very hard without you, my son.

I know that I will have to go on writing when I feel like this. The thoughts, memories, feelings come piling in. They overwhelm with their intensity. The only way I can make this burden lessen is to write it all out; to focus on you in a constructive way. I want to write about the things I loved about you. I want to write about all the good things you said about being able to spend your last weeks with us at home.

(Gabrielle)

We can see in this passage that despite the comfort she takes in his popularity, looking at photographs and watching videos, she 'can't get him out of her head'. She 'sees' him and 'hears' him and she turns to him for help to move on – to 'reclaim herself'. There is perhaps a paradox here, as she appears to feel her continued closeness to him is preventing her from moving on, yet it is to him she turns to release her.

Most of the accounts in this chapter are from parents whose son or daughter has died. However, even when their child survives, the emotional impact of the diagnosis and the knowledge that their son or daughter could die, continues to affect parents. Christine's son Tony had survived his illness, but she relates how hard it is to let him go having nearly lost him:

it's got worse now. No it's not got worse . . . His dad's actually gone to New Zealand so he's thinking about going out there now . . . he wants to go and I've got to sort of let him go, I've got to be, I've got to let him go, he's got his life. But you know, I think keep going back . . . Yeah with cancer you go through different stages, don't you, all you want to hear the doctor say is 'yeah he's in remission'. And then you come home but you're still going back every, I think it's every two weeks for check-ups, it's every so many weeks. So the first year after, even though Tony was in remission he's still got that pressure, that's why I couldn't go to work and I found it so difficult, and that's when I found it really, really hit me. It was the going back and the stress of it. I mean you just live for that thing, and then you live like for six weeks, and then you live for so many weeks, and I couldn't plan anything. I had to plan like the holiday was like, you know you just couldn't do that, you were just planning for week to week. You know somebody said 'oh we'll go away'. Oh no you can't, you've got to wait for this, and it's still like that now. It gets gradually worse, because the appointments, touch wood, are only six months. There's one due actually in a couple of weeks' time but the two weeks before . . . It's just the appointments and waiting for the results and going 'cause you are scared the week before . . . Really you are just like, in the first 12 months you sort of like you have about a week where you feel OK 'cause you are dreading going, say it's a six weeks appointment, you build yourself up to it to one week and then you don't get the results for another week, so that's two weeks gone. And then you've got like another four weeks to the next appointment and then you are dreading the next two weeks and it just goes on and on and on. And at the end of it, you know, you are just emotionally drained and I find it so hard . . . I mean you never, ever sleep, I mean you are just constantly there all the time. Even since, really it's only in the last 12 months that I've felt all right and that's just because I've gone back to work, took my mind off it. But it's there all the time.

(Christine)

Spiritual support

Some of the narratives mentioned religious beliefs and spirituality in relation to managing the bereavement process; some mention of this has already been made in George's story and in Charlotte's quotation. The following extracts all relate in some way to spirituality and the way in which it has helped – or not helped.

Charlotte's account suggests that her faith in God has been of fundamental importance to her:

I do have a spiritual belief that there is a God who cares for everyone and everything and that helped. At least two nurses said I was strong 'how do you cope?' and others said that too I said my spiritual beliefs helped . . . I had told my other children and their (and Sean's) friends that they should not be afraid of death (or life) or they would be insulting God who loves and cares for us all and all things.

(Charlotte)

George's mother, Helen, has told me that George's own spirituality increased as his physical strength decreased. His belief in God was a source of considerable comfort at the end of his life and a tape-recording of him telling Helen that he felt 'it was right to return to God at this point' was used at his funeral service. Denise C expresses a similar belief in the wisdom of God when reflecting on her own son Alexander's faith and that of George:

If only they had been able to meet – I wonder what they would have said? I do believe that our respective sons must have been so very special in God's eyes and that he hand-picked them for greater works. All children are special but it seems to me they possessed extra qualities which are not of earthly making . . . Alexander had been modestly ambitious in his career plans but simply said to me, 'God has other plans now for me'. I cry so much when I think back on those poignant moments of conversation . . .

(Denise C)

Again we see a greater power being honoured for events that cannot be understood in earthly 'rational' terms, and thus comfort is derived that these young men were in some way destined to die young in order to fulfill God's work.

Anne's belief in an after-life and the support from her church have helped her, as they have her daughter:

Another life-line for me has been my local church who have all been very supportive. I think my belief in after-life has got me through some very dark days. My youngest daughter, now 15, had also found some relief from her anguish by her religion. Her school has always been very supportive and understanding and helped her through the very difficult time of her brother's death when she was in her first year at High School. Many of her teachers had also known Chris and helped.

(Anne)

Again Geraldine's account tells us of the support a church can provide:

We all three had a lot of support from three churches in Norwich. The one where my husband and I are members had a number of prayer groups and two of these, where at least one member knew Katy and us well, prayed for us regularly and kept in touch with each step. The members of these groups still ask about each hospital appointment. The church where Katy was a member and the one where she had been a member also visited her/us and sent cards and flowers.

(Geraldine)

Claire, whose husband is a clergyman, acknowledges the help and support she has been given through the church:

> Although ultimately we were alone, we were greatly supported by a large and loving church congregation – my husband is a clergyman. I wonder how we would have managed without their love and support, alongside with that of our extended family. But the other dimension was that I felt that people were watching . . .
>
> (Claire)

Helen V acknowledges that spirituality was a support to Simon – as it was to Alexander. Although they had never needed to discuss such things before, his imminent death made it seem 'natural':

> I suppose values and beliefs are being consolidated in early adulthood. Simon sang in the Anglican cathedral until his voice broke, and then was no longer interested in the church. Be he had the idealism of youth. He admired the Dalai Lama, fasted for famine relief. When we realised death was near, it seemed natural to talk about what would happen after, though we'd never ever spoken of spiritual things before. It was too hard to say much once we'd started, but we just mused at times when he was in hospital. We didn't talk about the sort of funeral he should have. I hope he was able to talk to the nurses in the hospice about dying. I wish I could have done more of this. I've lost any attachment to organised religion myself – not all that pleased with God either.
>
> (Helen V)

However, Helen V in ending this passage by saying that she is 'not all that pleased with God' suggests that in contrast to other accounts, rather than finding solace in the church, she has lost her attachment to organized religion.

Sue also rejects religion:

> I wouldn't be averse to counselling as such, only unfortunately there is little available here [in Southern Germany] and what is on offer is always in the hands of the church, which as a non-believer, I find counter-productive.
>
> (Sue)

Here we see that while she may have considered counselling to be useful, this would not be acceptable if it were in the hands of the church.

A father's perspective

Thus far, mothers have written all the extracts in this chapter and most of those included in the book as a whole. The following two passages have, in contrast, been written by fathers and may shed some light on whether there is a fundamental difference between the ways in which men and women express their grief and response to the impact of the illness. First we hear from Luke whose son Martin survived testicular cancer:

> I am terrified of what they are going to do to him, and they are not even going to do it to me. Wish I knew how to do the best for him; can't just go on as though nothing is happening; can't keep talking about it because it is all that I think about; can't just huddle in mutual 'I love you dad' 'I love you son', got to have a good cry, better out than in, stuff – partly because such displays are against both our natures, requiring large doses of anti-emetics, and partly because I do not think it helps him to endure his lot.
>
> But does he feel supported by me? Trish gets so cross with anything I say to him. Paradoxically, I think he does know I am trying my best and actually feels sorry for me when I keep on getting it wrong. She of course, is tireless, steady as a rock, and Martin could not ask for a better companion in adversity.
>
> (Luke)

It is perhaps a very 'male' perspective, that while Luke wants at some level to cry and hug Martin, it is not possible for two men to display emotions in this way. As he says rather acerbically, such a display would require 'large doses of anti-emetics'. Luke would suffer instead of Martin if he could, but seems to doubt that Martin knows that he is supported by him. He feels he gets everything wrong, whilst in contrast he appears to feel that everything Martin's mother does is right. We have, however, seen accounts from mothers who also feel that they are failing, letting the family down and being a burden, thus Luke's feelings may be less gendered and more generalizable.

Michael's account relates the immense difficulty he has had in coming to terms with his son Miles's death:

> During those two long years of nursing my son, I had this terrible fear of becoming ill or somehow incapacitated myself, preventing me from attending him. Somehow I managed to find the inner resources to meet each dreadful day.
>
> Parents who have lost adult children in accidents I know will find it hard to appreciate the enormous sense of relief, and almost exhilaration when Miles died. He had suffered certainly as much as any human being ever has suffered, and it was suddenly very wonderful to know that he would suffer no more.
>
> This feeling (also shared by my wife) lasted about two months, before depression set in – a depression that has not left me since.
>
> Each day I am haunted, not so much by his death, but by his tragic life. Despite the fact that he is no longer suffering, the slightest thing

can trigger off in my mind some event or circumstance of those two long years, and send me spiralling downwards. Miles is always in my thoughts. If one sees life as a TV screen, then those traumatic events occupy 65% of that screen.

I feel the average person is completely unable to appreciate what losing a child is like. I am inclined to lose my temper when people say (and so many do) – 'I know just what it's like, I lost my old dad last year – he was 92!' I am only really at ease when in the company of similar parents (with the group 'Compassionate Friends' for instance).

If I ever had a fear of death (I can't remember) I certainly have no such fear now. I tend to live life for the present, as one never knows what is round the corner. I tend never to think about the past, that is, the years before my son became ill; I guess it is because I was living with a time bomb. I can no longer read a book. I dread bed-time each night, as I can never get to sleep, and when I do, it is never for more than two hours.

In my mental healing process, I know one day I will have to deal with my son's death. Meanwhile it is as much as I can do to deal with the memory of his tragic life.

If a doctor came to me and said, 'just take these tablets and your grief will go away', I know there is no way I would take that treatment – I know that I need my grief as much as I need air to breath.

(Michael)

Michael's narrative has much in common with those written by mothers. He speaks of the same irritation at well-meaning people who say they know how he feels when they compare the loss of an elderly relative. He also says he is only at ease in the company of other parents who have also had a similar experience. In common with Charlotte, Michael can no longer read a book. Although this is not documented in George's mother's account, I know it to be true of her as I once lent her a novel by a favourite author which she politely accepted, but later admitted she would be unable to read. In common with George's mother, Michael says that during Miles's illness he feared that he would be incapacitated by illness himself. So physical was Helen's response to the stress of George's illness that she feared her own death would pre-date George's. However, for both Michael and Helen the prospect of their own deaths now that their sons have died, no longer appears terrifying. Michael also tells us that he cannot sleep and suffers from depression, but in the final sentence we see that he says that he needs his grief as much as he needs the air to breath. This suggests a need to stay close to the pain and the loss in a way that challenges the notion of 'moving on' through a linear progression towards recovery.

These last two extracts from Luke and Michael seem to suggest that there is little difference in the way that grief and pain affect men and women. The ability to express it may differ, but the internal processes have much in common. It may, however, be more difficult for men to express their grief in a society where a man's emotional reaction is expected to remain private. Men are expected to be strong (as we saw in the first chapter) and men's tears may be a cause of embarrassment in a way in which women's are not.

Reflections

This has probably been the most difficult chapter to write, it may also be the most difficult to read. It is full of pain, anguish and grief, and the parents speak volumes about their experience in a way that communicates itself to the reader more powerfully than any academic or theoretical analysis. It is thus difficult to comment on the narratives without being in danger of slipping into 'trite' or 'banal' observations that add little to the evidence already presented. Indeed it has been clearly established through the narratives that no one who has not experienced the death of a child can truly understand – nevertheless, I will try at this point to reflect on some of the issues raised.

We can see from these narratives that while, predictably, immense pain is apparent in every case, the parents seek and on occasions find comfort in different ways. Some find support through continued contact or volunteer work with the hospices where their children have been cared for, others seek support from families who have experienced similar problems. Others seek 'normality'. Yet these needs may change across time, between different people and between couples; neither are they linear. Rather, there are signs of 'progress' interspersed by many relapses. Some parents have even found the passing of time and distance problematic in that they feel a separation from their lost child, and expectations that they should have 'moved on' prove unrealistic. The phrase 'roller coaster of emotions' has been used by several of the respondents throughout the book, and this seems significant.

Many of the parents have spoken about the impossibility of anyone who has not experienced the death or life-threatening illness of a child understanding their pain. Rosenblatt (2000b), through an analysis of narratives from bereaved parents, identifies this phenomenon as a 'chasm' between bereaved parents and other people. He suggests that there is an assumption by others that parents will get over their grief quickly and that this lack of understanding helps to maintain the chasm. Bereaved parents, according to Rosenblatt, are engulfed by devastating feelings that make everyone who does not share those feelings seem distant and uncaring. We have seen this phenomenon addressed repeatedly through the narratives in this chapter.

The narratives also suggest that spirituality has been of enormous help to some respondents, whilst others have felt anger with a God who could allow such pain and loss. Such differential responses are also documented by Rosenblatt (2000b), who cites narratives from parents who have felt that God has helped them to find peace, meaning and hope. One respondent said that you could still be angry with God whilst keeping your faith (2000a: 216). However, in contrast, many parents' narratives in Rosenblatt's book dealt with the challenge the death had posed to their religious beliefs. They could not believe that a God who was just, wise, compassionate and all-powerful, could allow their child to die. As we can see Rosenblatt's work in this area (2000a, 2000b) has covered many of the same issues and made similar observations, unrelated to the age of the lost child.

The reader of this book might ask 'what has this chapter to do with life stage?' After all, the difficulties, emotions, pain and anguish expressed by the respondents in this chapter might apply to the loss of a child at any age. The question of whether there is a 'less heartbreaking time for a child to die' has already been asked (see Chapter 1) and the answer is 'no'. However, what the preceding chapters have established is that the parents of young adults with cancer face some quite specific problems.

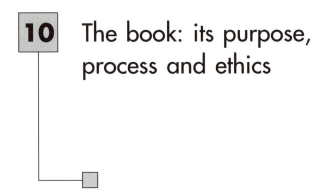

10 The book: its purpose, process and ethics

The final chapter in this book posed something of a dilemma. Should it try to sum up all that precedes it? Should it attempt to offer a theoretical interpretation? Should it make recommendations for policy and practice? None of these options seemed a suitable conclusion to the immediacy and rawness of the material contained thus far. There are no neat conclusions, and no summary can assure the reader of the value of a particular course of action. It therefore seemed more appropriate to conclude with a reflection on the process, on my part within it and to include also Helen and Geoff's reactions. Helen's contribution to this chapter comes first, Geoff's second and mine ends both the chapter and the book.

'Connections' – Helen's need for continuity and for activity related to George

This book arose from my most profound need to take George with me into a future, which would no longer contain his physical presence, and for activity, which connected me with him. I was very ill for several months immediately after George died and so it was some time before I was able to find enough energy to work out exactly what I should do but once I felt better I can honestly say that the book found me.

The word 'effortless' keeps recurring when I look back over the two years since I first went to talk to George's Lancaster oncologist, Professor McIllmurray, about our ideas for a research project into young adults and cancer. Of course it hasn't been 'easy' at all, but on some level the research, once started, has had a life of its own and it has felt as if we have simply been the catalysts for something that was waiting to be published. Indeed much of the book had already been written by other parents before this project was launched – in diaries, poems, letters, in private notebooks. All that was required was some way of finding these individual stories and then combining them into one 'meta-story'. I don't think that I ever really doubted that other stories would confirm what we already knew at a personal level, that young adults with cancer and their parents have to cope with difficulties specific to their life stage as well as with their illness. What has surprised me, however, is that this book has not been written before.

Reflecting back now on how quickly this book has come about since Geoff and I first talked over the possibility of a research project in the autumn of 1999 I think that the most difficult obstacle we had to overcome was the belief that actually this research and this book must already exist and that somehow we hadn't been able to find it. The task of convincing ourselves that we weren't duplicating work that had been done elsewhere went on even after we had sent out our appeal for other parents' stories. We didn't become fully convinced that there really was a serious gap in information until the first letters and phone calls began to arrive at the university and we discovered that other parents felt the same.

I don't think that Geoff will mind my saying that in the early days of this project he took a back seat. Our responses to grief are different, I need activity and contact with people and lots of opportunity to talk about my feelings, Geoff needs quiet, personal space and solitary walks. The original suggestion of a research project came from Geoff but the determination to get it off the ground and the need to immerse myself in 'George related' activities were mine and in many ways it was very therapeutic for me to do so. For four years every waking moment had been devoted to the well-being of George and the rest of the family. I had no desire at all to fill the now empty moments with anything that wasn't connected with him so to be able to engage in this research was a lifeline.

Once the hurdle of whether to proceed was cleared and we were put in touch with Anne Grinyer and Carol Thomas as possible researchers I began to feel a lot more confident. More importantly, suddenly and miraculously we discovered that there were now four people committed to the research and that we had found two women who were going to take much of the burden from us. It was at this point that we found our direction and the project became more than just an idea and began to take shape.

Carol's contribution was critical in determining the shape and direction the research should take and in finding an approach that would allow parents' voices to be heard. We knew that we wanted to hear what other parents of young adults with cancer had to say about what they had found (or were still finding) to be the key issues for this age group. But we also knew that we mustn't influence their answers by coming up with our own list of what we had found to be significant. Furthermore, we knew that participation in the research had to be absolutely voluntary, being aware at first hand how painful it can be to recall the experiences of the anguish and helplessness of accompanying a young adult child on their cancer journey. Carol's willingness to be involved was crucial, she had experience of research into the social impacts of cancer on individuals and families and had already worked with 'Prof Mac'. She had also successfully used the narrative form of research in order to look at women and disability. She was therefore confident that if we simply disseminated an appeal for personal stories through charities, hospices and local newspapers we would get the responses we were looking for but with all the contributions given freely and without any pressure. Undertaking the task of appealing for personal accounts, of writing to organizations and of networking generally was exactly the sort of activity I knew I could manage. It gave me just what I needed, plenty to do which connected me with George.

Once the project was off the ground, however, and the narratives began to arrive on Anne and Carol's desks at the Institute for Health Research there was a period of several months when we very much left it all to them. I was back at work and couldn't sustain the level of activity without a break. It was actually a great relief to feel that the research was now underway and in safe hands and that we had started something that no longer needed my full attention. We were still very newly bereaved and found that it was too distressing to read the narratives but Anne let us know when she and Carol had been contacted by other parents and passed on letters addressed to us. The letters were wonderful and so encouraging, letting us know that this book really had to be published and thanking us for giving other parents the chance to be heard and to pay tribute to their children. Several of the parents have remained in regular contact, giving enormous support. Some of them are involved in similar work of their own. Carol is a counsellor specializing in work with young adult cancer patients. Sue has just written the biography of Alex's fight against osteosarcoma and we compare notes by email at least once a week. Carol S took Anne and I round Martin House Children's Hospice where she is involved with the appeal to build a new unit for young adults.

In very many ways I feel that there has been an inevitability about the publication of this book. Even in the short time since we appealed to parents to send us their stories there has been an increased awareness of the special needs of young adults. But I know that without Anne as author and without her incredible empathy with the subject matter it would have been very difficult to produce something so sensitive to our original intention to give parents a voice. The fact that Professor Tony Gatrell's (Institute for Health Research) suggestion that she might be interested in this research was made without the knowledge that she had known George since he was a baby, is only one of many coincidences we have encountered along the way. Probably it would have been difficult for her to refuse. It has been very hard on her at times. Not only has she immersed herself in the stories she has also spent hours listening to me talk about George and about his illness so that she could understand exactly what matters to parents supporting a young adult with cancer. As the research proceeded I realized more and more that I could share my memories and feelings with Anne and that she would be able to weave them together with the stories from all the other parents into one cohesive whole, which would do justice to our amazing children and to the love we feel for them. The way she has managed to order so many words and so much pain without diminishing the power of parents' writings has surpassed our greatest expectations and we are so pleased that she agreed to get involved and particularly that she has been willing to follow where the stories have led.

Geoff's reflections

Helen has written that this was a book waiting to be written. Another way of looking at it is that it has been the result of a number of lucky coincidences. Whilst some are obvious from what Helen has written, others are more personal and there are one or two of these that I want to explore here. I teach and research in a Management School and have done so for nearly 30 years. Therefore it was not surprising, when we were thinking about how to fulfil George's wish to help people in the situation that we had all endured for four years, that I suggested we do some research.

Of course we had already begun the process even when George was alive. We did the normal thing of trying to find out what had been written about the cancer and its impact on patients and those close to them. What did rather surprise me was that the books and articles I read that were most helpful were those written not by doctors or researchers or academics but by people who had gone through similar experiences to our own. So when Carol and Anne suggested that the research should involve collecting and analysing the 'stories' of parents like us I was pleased. I felt that the nature of parents' experiences were more likely to persuade them to 'tell it like it was and is' for them.

I was reinforced in my views about the research method Anne and Carol adopted when I began to look at what research had already been done in the area of peoples' responses to cancer diagnosis and treatment. The vast majority of research was done using questionnaires with the replies having to fit into categories determined by the researchers allowing the respondents little freedom to express their own views or feelings. To do so makes massive assumptions about how people are thinking and feeling. In addition it seems to me to be verging on the unethical, for example, to ask someone undergoing chemotherapy to tick boxes as a way of gauging what they are experiencing.

The choice of research method was fully justified by the quality of the responses. They were all we could have asked for and more. They were inspiring, humbling, insightful, enormously sad and, very occasionally, unexpectedly funny. But above all they spoke about the humanity and courage of those who wrote. I know we all cried whilst reading them. Even now I know that re-reading certain sentences can still move me to tears. And that is how it should be. The experience of having a young adult child fall ill with cancer can only be communicated by evoking the emotions as well as logic. It should involve feelings as well as numbers.

Over the years I have come to a particular view about research and its relationship to the audiences it might have. First, it seems to me that we have to combine what some would call 'objective' research with 'subjective'. But currently, in most fields and especially in health research, the balance is almost always in favour of the former. This imbalance needs to be addressed but the barriers to change are high.

Second, if you want to make a difference then you have to reach your intended audience. You can do this using the right medium and the right message. I am sure that this book has the right message. It is a powerful statement about what it is to be a parent of a young adult child with cancer. There will be, I believe, a very short distance between the writers and the reader. I have some reservations about the medium. Books have a certain kind of audience. It is to be hoped that professionals will read it because they are professionals. I am sure that some parents who are in the situation that Helen and I are in will read it. But some won't and I think we need to try to get to that audience by different means. However, I am comforted by the fact that George loved books and relied on them to get him through some of the worst times. It is fitting that he features so prominently in the one he has inspired.

Finally, I would just like to say how much I have learned, mostly standing on the sidelines but sometimes on the pitch, watching the book emerge. The research process has been quite unlike any I have experienced. It concerns, in the most intimate way, what Helen and I have been through in the past few years. It isn't out there but in here. Has it been cathartic? Not in the sense that most people would mean. I don't agree with the idea that we all go through the same grieving or coping processes. And I believe that one thing that comes out strongly from the research is that people deal with the same situation in different ways. The book has helped but I would be hard put to describe exactly how. But perhaps I don't need to.

The research and writing the book has involved people to whom I am very close and has naturally spilled over in to my personal life more than I have experienced before. It has been very rewarding but also demanding. It has, however, been especially gratifying to watch a gifted, sensitive and professional researcher and writer at work. Anne has done an excellent job, very quickly, despite having to work closely with two of her research subjects! Without her the project could never have got off the ground and Helen and I are both very grateful to her.

Endings – Anne's personal reflections on the book

I have over the years been involved in a number of research projects and have subsequently published accounts of their findings, but my involvement in 'George's' research has proved to be a very different experience on many levels. At the beginning of any research process there are concerns that the research may fail to answer the question adequately, that respondents will not be found or that publication will prove problematic, and George's project was no different in that all those concerns applied. However, in addition, I was also acutely aware of the responsibility I had accepted in attempting to fulfill George's parents' hopes for the research and its outcome. The research project was a tribute to their lost son, undertaken in order to help other families and funded by a charitable trust set up in George's memory. The fund had been generated by donations from friends and family and through the efforts of many of George's friends, who had undertaken sponsored events to raise money. It is a tribute to George that he continues to be remembered in this way. His parents are still receiving donations from young people they hardly know, but who remember George.

So, many hopes and expectations were invested in the successful outcome of the research. Additionally, I have been a friend of George's family for nearly 30 years, thus the success of the project was important to me at a more personal level than is usually the case. In the 'publish or perish' culture of academia in the twenty-first century, research and publication dominate academic life. However, if this project failed the implications were, for me, more far-reaching than career-related considerations. I would have felt that I had let down George's family, his friends and George himself, as before he died he indicated his wish that his parents should do something to help other young adults and their families travelling together on the cancer journey. For all these reasons I was uncertain about the wisdom of taking on the research. How glad I am that I took the risk, for this research and its outcome has been the most rewarding of experiences. The process has in many ways been very challenging, it has been distressing and it has been painful, but it has also given me an insight into the courage of the many young people and their parents whose stories are told in this book, and has revealed the enduring nature of the parent–child bond and the importance of love. It has been a privilege to share a small part of the cancer journey with those who have trusted me with their experiences.

The responsibility I feel towards George's family is extended to all the contributors to the book. The appeal for narratives written by George's mother, Helen, resulted in contributing parents addressing what was probably the most painful experience of their lives, in most cases committing it to paper and finally entrusting this most personal and intimate account to a complete stranger. The justification for such a method is that it gives a voice to those whose experiences would otherwise remain undocumented and unheard. Yet there is an ever present danger of exploitation, of taking the lived and often painful experiences of vulnerable people and using them for the advancement of an academic career or for the benefit of others involved in the research and publication process. I was mindful throughout of these issues and have tried to act with integrity and sensitivity towards those people whose stories have been told in this book.

The need to act in such a way has thrown up a number of initially unanticipated problems relating to the treatment of the data. In the early stages of the data collection phase I felt a strong impulse to allow the narratives to be presented in their entirety and was resistant to using them instrumentally by extracting quotations to illustrate particular issues. However, given the sheer volume of narrative material generated – in excess of 130,000 words – and a much more practical and realistic stance from the editor, it became apparent that to use the narratives in their entirety would be impossible. A book based on such an approach would have been much too lengthy – some narratives were in excess of 50 pages – and would also have been difficult to read. This left me with the challenge of doing justice to the material – and its authors – whilst at the same time acknowledging that the majority of the narrative material would not be published.

Bearing in mind these considerations, I set about the process of synthesizing the data. There is a reflection on the analysis of the narratives in the methodological discussion included at the end of the first chapter, but it is not the technical and academic process that I want to consider further here. Rather, it is the way in which I attempted to treat the material with respect, maintaining its integrity and honouring its authors whilst at the same time, through necessity, fragmenting it. This process was also made more problematic because some of the narratives lent themselves to having extracts taken from them to illustrate thematic issues much more readily than others. Indeed some writers had already done the 'thematic analysis' for me and had written under headings that correspond closely with the chapters' themes. But other narratives, no less insightful or relevant, were much more akin to outpourings of grief and pain, unstructured and difficult to use in an instrumental fashion. I have used extracts from these narratives, in fact all those who contributed to the project are represented in the text, but the difference in the approach and style of the contributors has led to a discrepancy in the number of times a given respondent is cited. Despite this, all the narratives were invaluable to the research, all were carefully read and all contributed to the foundations that underpin the book. In addition, I shed many tears over the narrative material. Each time a new narrative was received I had to brace myself for the pain I would encounter in its pages.

I remember answering the telephone to a colleague whilst reading a newly arrived narrative. I must have sounded upset because she asked me what was the matter. I told her about the task I was engaged in and how difficult it was to read accounts of pain and grief so movingly told by parents. To illustrate this I attempted to read a few lines to her, I could not; my tears would not allow me.

The justification for this process, for expecting parents to share their experiences and for representing those experiences as honorably as I can, is that the book is designed to be of use. Unlike much academic work, which remains obscure and dusty on library shelves or which is read and cited only by other academics, I hope that this book will make a difference to the lives of those who read it. During the writing process I showed chapters to a variety of interested parties who read the material from a number of different perspectives. Health professionals, academics, friends of George's family and members of George's family have all read some or all of the text, and all have commented on the different ways it can be read. Indeed, all appear to have taken different things from the text.

Health professionals will, I hope, find the book useful in their professional practice utilizing the material to reassure parents, but may also recommend it, as appropriate, to parents coping with the problems discussed. The 'reflections' and suggestions on the implications for health professionals at the end of each chapter are designed to be of practical use. The parents and families of young adults with cancer will also, I hope, find the book of use in contextualizing their experiences. The organization of the book allows for the reader to be easily directed to issues of relevance, but beyond this thematic organization, the book can also be read at different levels. For example, some readers may want to read only the narrative material, or to track through George's story at the start of each chapter, others may instead prefer to leave aside the narrative data and read only the commentary on it or the reflections at the ends of the chapters. An academic audience teaching about or researching related issues may also find the book of use. For them not only the empirical material, but also the synthesis of others' studies in Chapter 1, may be of interest. Throughout the preparation of this book those who have read drafts at various stages have commented on the flexibility of the book, each of them focusing on different aspects and taking different meanings according to their relationship to the material.

The role of George's mother Helen cannot be overstated, she has played an active role since the inception of the process, and without her appeal as a bereaved parent it is unlikely that so many narratives would have been submitted. She has also been in correspondence with all of the contributing parents on a number of occasions. The importance of maintaining contact with the parents has been a crucial part of the attempt to maintain an ethical stance towards the narrative material and its authors. At each stage of the process the respondents have been kept informed by Helen of progress, consulted on how they and their family would like to be represented and sent material such as the journal publication based on the narratives (Grinyer and Thomas 2001a). Helen has also been brave enough to reflect on the painful memories of her experience of George's illness and death. The introductions to each chapter are the result of a taped interview with me. A difficult experience for us both, which had to be done in several sittings and which left us both feeling drained and emotional.

George's father, Geoff, has also been closely involved in the writing process. As an academic he has much experience of research and publication and I have valued his opinion throughout, though at times, particularly in the early stages, I found it difficult to expose my work to his scrutiny as an academic, as George's father and as a friend. Again the role confusion of being both friend and professional created an additional and challenging dimension to the research.

So the process of writing this book has been an emotional and painful one at a number of levels: because of my relationship with George's family, because of my fondness for George and because the narratives were so moving. But I am acutely aware that however painful the process has been for me, it bears no comparison to the pain endured by parents who have watched their children's lives destroyed by cancer. I am the parent of two young adult sons who have thankfully never been diagnosed with life-threatening illness, I can only imagine how I would feel if they were. Nevertheless, in every account I read I could not help thinking that this could have been my Tom or Ben and wondering, if it were, if I would be able to find the courage shown by the parents in this book.

Although my name is on the cover of this book as the author, I share authorship with all those whose stories are told within its pages.

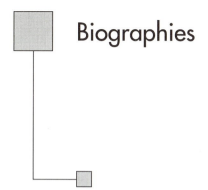

Biographies

The following biographies are for reference to remind the reader of the relevant characteristics of the respondents and their children. They are listed under the name of the parent, as it is they who are quoted in the text. Readers will notice that some first names are replicated, that is because some respondents wished their own names to be used and more than one person of the same name contributed a narrative or had a child of the same name. Where this is the case with the contributing parent, an initial is included after the first name for ease of identification. Where it is their son or daughter who has the same name as another young adult (as in the case of Laura, Simon and Michael) their identity is also indicated by an initial after the name of one of them.

Anne, a doctor, also married to a doctor and mother of **Christopher** and his three sisters. Christopher was diagnosed with chronic myeloid leukaemia when he was 20 and about to start at university. He died when he was 21.

Barbara, mother of **Jamie** and his younger brother. Jamie survived Hodgkin's disease, which was diagnosed at the age of 18 when he was a student.

Brenda, married to **Michael** and mother of Amanda, Lisa and **Miles**. Miles died from neuroblastoma, which was diagnosed at the age of 23. He was ill for two years. His girlfriend was called Polly. Brenda and Michael sent in joint accounts.

Candy, mother of Bethany and of **Sianne**. Sianne died from rhabdo-myosarcoma, which she developed three years after her father had com-mitted suicide. Candy's older children had left home at this time.

Carol S, mother of Paul and of **J** who died from osteosarcoma when he was a student.

Carol, mother of **Sara** who died from non-Hodgkin's lymphoma at the age of 25 after being ill for 14 months.

Charlotte, mother of Ian, Angus, Serena and of **Sean.** Sean died from osteosarcoma diagnosed at the age of 17.

Christine, single parent and mother of **Tony** who survived teratoma diagnosed when he was 15. Unlike the narrative material from other contributors, which was written by them, extracts from Christine's story are based on an interview between her and the author. Thus her contribution has a more 'spoken' quality than the other narrative passages.

Claire, mother of **Laura W** who died from a brain tumour at the age of 21. She is married to Jeffry and is also the mother of Eleanor, and twins Gregory and Luke.

Denise, mother of **Laura** and Philip and married to Colin. Laura was diagnosed with osteosarcoma when she was 15; she died four years later.

Denise C, married to Phil and mother of **Alexander** and Ben. Alexander died from rhabdomyosarcoma, aged 21, whilst he was a student.

Donald and Annie, parents of **Donna** who survived acute lymphoblastic leukaemia, and of **Felicity** who survived Hodgkin's disease. Both girls were at school at the time of their diagnoses.

Elizabeth, single parent and mother of John and **Michael T.** Michael died from osteosarcoma diagnosed when he was 15, he was ill for three years.

Gabrielle, married to Richard and mother of Kate and **Steve.** Steve died when he was 24. Extracts from Gabrielle's narrative are taken from her letters to Steve written after his death from melanoma.

Geraldine, mother of **Katy** who survived ovarian cancer. She was diagnosed when she was 19 and was a student at the time.

Helen, married to Geoff and mother of Jonathan, **George** and David. George died from osteosarcoma at the age of 23 having been ill for four years. He was a student at the time of his diagnosis.

Helen V, living in Australia, married to Patrick and mother of two daughters – one of whom, Sarah, was at university at the time of diagnosis – and of **Simon.** Simon died from a kidney tumour four weeks after diagnosis at the age of 19, having travelled from Australia to London. He was a student at the time of his diagnosis.

Iris, married to Geoff and mother of Nathan, Sacha and **Matthew.** Matthew died from Ewing's sarcoma first diagnosed when he was 12; he was ill for nine years.

Jean, married to Brian and mother of **Susan**. Susan was married, had a son and died from a brain tumour at the age of 28.

Jeremy and **Lesley,** parents of Daniel, Edward and **Timothy**. Timothy survived testicular cancer diagnosed when he was a student aged 21.

Joyce, mother of **Jill** and two other daughters. Jill died from osteosarcoma when she was 24, she had been ill for 20 months.

Luke, married to Trish and father of Ida and **Martin**. Martin survived testicular cancer that was diagnosed when he was 22 and, at the time of writing, is about to marry Sophie.

Lynn, married to Ray and mother of Manda, Cindy and **Simon R**. Simon died at the age of 21 from choriocarcinoma that was diagnosed 20 months earlier. His girlfriend's name was Jody. Extracts from Lynn's narrative are taken from 'Modern Life is Rubbish', a journal of Simon's illness written by Lynn as a tribute to his courage.

Mary, mother of **Nicola**. Nicola died from malignant melanoma diagnosed when she was 15 years old. She died when she was 22; she was a student at the time.

Moira, married to Bill and mother of **Alasdair** and a younger son. Alasdair died from osteosarcoma at the age of 19. He had been ill for four years and was a student at the time of his death.

Sue, living in Germany, married to Wolfgang and mother of Natalie, Benjamin and **Alex**. Alex died from osteosarcoma at the age of 22 after being ill for two years. Sue was a co-founder of an informal support group for parents of young adults with cancer.

Sue B, married to Mike and mother of Jacqui and **Paul**. Paul died from Hodgkin's disease; he was ill for five years and was 26 when he died. Paul married Teresa during the year before his death. The extracts from Sue B's narrative are taken from a diary she wrote during Paul's illness.

Note

The process of fulfilling respondents' wishes in relation to the use of real names or pseudonyms has been very complex as many of the transcripts were originally allocated pseudonyms to protect identities. However, after consultation, the majority of parents wished their own and their children's real names to be used, thus all names in these transcripts had to be changed. Conversely some of those transcripts not allocated pseudonyms belonged to parents who wished their identities to remain anonymous. Coupled with this some of the early pseud-onyms allocated were the real names of subsequent respondents, again necessitating changes. Every care has been taken during the editing of the book to ensure that parents' preferences have been accurately represented in the text and many hours have been spent checking and rechecking. It is however a concern that an inappropriate name will have slipped through, if this is the case please accept my apologies.

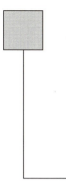

Appendix: Examples of the calls for narratives

Letter to organizations

Dear Sir or Madam,

We wonder whether there is any way in which your organisation could help us with our appeal for personal stories from parents who have experienced cancer in a son or daughter when their 'child' was a young adult?

The enclosed press release explains the origin of the project and we would be most grateful if you could publicize it via any newsletter, notice board, meeting, conference, etc. to which you have access. We are approaching all UK hospices in the hope that they can reach possible respondents via their newsletters and bereavement services and also hope to have something published in national media.

We have been very fortunate in that colleagues in the health and academic professions have freely given of their time and expertise. As a result of these discussions we have become convinced that there is a gap in both knowledge and support for parents of young adults with cancer.

Our ultimate goal is to find some way of supporting these parents, especially while their 'child' is terminally ill. In the first instance, however, we need to find out more about other parents' experiences, hence this request in the hope that you can assist.

Thank you.

Yours faithfully

Press release

Lancaster University research – How parents deal with a young adult's cancer.

Cancer in young adults, and its effects on parents, is the subject of a research project being launched by Lancaster University's Institute for Health Research. The research is being carried out in memory of George, who was treated for bone cancer at the Royal Orthopaedic and Heartlands hospitals in Birmingham but later died.

As part of the project the researchers would like to hear from parents who have had first-hand experience of supporting a child, in the 18–25 age range, through cancer. By means of these real-life accounts the research team hopes to identify particular problems and issues that arise when parents undergo this demanding ordeal.

All personal accounts will be in strictest confidence and no names will be used in publication.

The researchers hope that the research will lead to publications that will provide help and information for parents and professionals working in the field of teenage and young person cancer.

If you would like to take part in the study please send a written account or tape-recording to:

Caring through Cancer Project,
The Institute for Health Research,
Lancaster University,
Lancaster LA1 4YT.

For further information on the project contact Dr Anne Grinyer or Dr Carol Thomas.

Press release

Can you help us with our research project into young adult cancer sufferers and the effect of their illness on their families, especially parents?

Geoff and Helen's middle son **George** died in March 1999 after a four-year battle against osteosarcoma (bone cancer), which was diagnosed when he was a first-year student at Sheffield University. He was 19 when the tumour in his right leg was discovered and 23 when he died. His treatment at the Royal Orthopaedic Hospital in Birmingham and at the Royal Lancaster Infirmary (his home hospital) was superb and his approach courageous in the extreme. However, Geoff and Helen at times found the strain of supporting him overwhelming and feel that there are issues about George's stage of life which made their task as parents particularly hard.

As a result of their experience Geoff and Helen have decided to use money given in George's memory to fund a research project into the impact of cancer in a young adult, on their families, especially parents. This research will be undertaken at the Institute of Health Research at Lancaster University. As part of this research they would like to hear from others who have had first-hand experience of supporting (and possibly losing) a child, in the 18–25 age range, through cancer. By means of real-life accounts the research team hopes to identify particular problems and issues which arise when a young adult is suffering from cancer.

If you would like to take part in this study **would you send either a written account or a tape recording of your spoken account to Geoff and Helen at the address below.** You can make your account as long or short as you like, focusing on the problems and issues that you and your child faced during your child's illness. These personal accounts will be handled in the strictest confidence and in drawing on them for publication purposes no names or identifying details will be used. This 'real-life stories' approach to social research is proving to be very powerful and allows people to speak for themselves. George's parents hope that knowledge gained in this way will be of help to all those caught up in the devastating situation of a seriously ill young adult. They feel that it would have been enormously helpful for them, while they were supporting George, to read the experiences of other parents. They hope that a publication resulting from the research might find its way to others in the same situation in the future as well as providing information for professionals working in the field of teenage and young person cancer.

The researchers involved are:

Dr Anne Grinyer
Dr Carol Thomas
Please give either of them a ring or email them if you would like to know any more about the research.

Bibliography

Anderson, M. (2000) *Death in the Family*, Newcastle Centre for Family Studies, http://www.nc.ac.uk/ncts/document55.html (accessed 13 April 2000).

Apter, T. (2001) *The Myth of Maturity: what teenagers need from parents to become adults*. New York: W.W. Norton.

Baldwin, S. (1985) *The Costs of Caring, Families with Disabled Children*. London: Routledge and Kegan Paul.

Baumrucker, S. (2001) Medical marijuana, *American Journal of Hospice and Palliative Care*, 18(4): 227–8.

Belshaw. S. (1999) *Fly With a Miracle*. London: Denor Press.

Bennett, F. and Abrahams, C. (1994) *Unequal Opportunities: Children with Disabilities and Their Families Speak Out*. London: NCH Action for Children.

Beresford, B. (1995) *Expert Opinions: A National Survey of Parents Caring for a Severely Disabled Child*. Bristol: Policy Press.

Bone, M. and Meltzer, H. (1989) *The Prevalence of Disability Among Children, Report 3, OPCS Survey of Disability in Great Britain*. London: HMSO.

Borg, T. (1999) Cancer and its consequences on sexuality, *European Cancer Conference Abstract Book (ECCO 10)*, 12–16 September, Vienna, Austria, p. 29.

Brabant, S., Forsythe, C. and McFarlain, G. (1994) Defining the family after the death of a child, *Death Studies*, 18: 197–206.

Brannen, J., Dodd, K., Oakley, A. and Storey, P. (1994) *Young People, Health and Family Life*. Buckingham: Open University Press.

Cain, A., Fast, I. and Erikson, M. (1964) Children's disturbed reactions to the death of a sibling, *American Journal of Orthopsychiatry*, 34(4): 741–52.

Carter, G.T. and Rosen, B.S. (2001) Marijuana in the management of amyotrophic lateral sclerosis, *American Journal of Hospice and Palliative Care*, 18(4): 264–70.

Clark, D. and Seymour, J. (1999) *Reflections on Palliative Care*. Buckingham: Open University Press.

Corden, A., Sainsbury, R. and Sloper, P. (2001) *Financial Implications of the Death of a Child*. London: Family Policy Studies Centre.

Costain Schou, K. and Hewison, J. (1999) *Experiencing Cancer*. Buckingham: Open University Press.

Coxon, K. (2001) A sick joke, *Guardian Education*, 27 February, p. 10.

Department of Health (1995) [The Calman-Hine Report] *A Policy Framework for Commissioning Cancer Services: A Report by the Expert Advisory Group on Cancer to the Chief Medical Officers of England and Wales*. London: HMSO

Department of Health (2000) *The NHS Cancer Plan*. London: HMSO.

De Valck, C., Bensing, J. and Bruynooghe, R. (2001) Medical students' attitudes towards breaking bad news: an empirical test of the World Health Organization Model, *Psycho-Oncology*, 10(5): 398–409.

Dobson, B. and Middleton, S. (1998) *Paying to Care: The Cost of Childhood Disability*. York: Joseph Rowntree Foundation.

Donovan, K. (1993) Breaking bad news, in *Communicating Bad News: Behavioural Science Learning Modules*. Geneva: World Health Organization: 3–14.

Fallowfield, L. (1995) Psychosocial interventions in cancer. *British Medical Journal*, 311: 1316–17.

Fawzy, F.I., Fawzy, N.W., Arndt, L.A. and Pasnau, R.O. (1995) Critical review of psychosocial interventions in cancer care. *Archives of General Psychiatry*, 52(2): 100–113.

Field, D. (1989) *Nursing the Dying*. London: Tavistock/Routledge.

Field, D., Hockey, J. and Small, N. (eds) (1997) *Death, Gender and Ethnicity*. London: Routledge.

Frank, A.W. (1997) *The Wounded Storyteller*. Chicago, IL: University of Chicago Press.

Garmezy, N. (1985) Stress resistant children: the search for protective factors, in J.E. Stevenson (ed.) *Recent Research in Developmental Psychopathology*.Oxford: Pergamon.

Giddens, A. (1991) *Modernity and Self-identity: Self and Society in the Late Modern Age*. Cambridge: Polity.

Gilbert, K.R. (1996) We've had the same loss, why don't we have the same grief? Loss and differential grief in families, *Death Studies*, 20: 269–83.

Glaser, B. and Strauss, A. (1965) *Awareness of Dying*. Chicago, IL: Aldine.

Grinyer, A. and Thomas, C. (2001a) Young adults with cancer: The effect on parents and families, *The International Journal of Palliative Nursing*, 7(4): 162–70.

Grinyer, A. and Thomas, C. (2001b) Young Adults and Life-stage Issues: the effects [of cancer] on parents and families. Paper presented at The Second International Conference on Teenage Cancer and The Adolescent, Royal College of Physicians, London, March.

Hall, J.A. and Roter, D.L. (1998) Medical communication and gender: a summary of research, *Journal of Gender-Specific Medicine*, 1: 39–42.

Hautamaki, K. and Nojonen, K. (2001) Attitudes towards discussion about sexuality related issues with patients, *European Cancer Conference Abstract Book (ECCO 11)*, 21–25 October, Lisbon, p. 391.

Her Majesty's Government (1969) *The Family Law Reform Act 1969* (c.46), section 8.

Hunt, M. (1991) The identification and provision of care for the terminally ill at home by 'family' members, *Sociology of Health and Illness*, 13: 375–95.

Lynam, J. (1995) Supporting one another: the nature of family work when a young adult has cancer, *Journal of Advanced Nursing*, 22: 116–25.

Meyerowitz, B. (2001) *Sexuality and Cancer: the Personal and the Interpersonal*, http://cancerresources.mednet.ucla.edu/5_info5c_archive_lec/5c03_sexuality.htm (accessed 4 Dec 2001).

Miles, M.B. and Huberman, A.M. (1994) *Qualitative Data Analysis*. London: Sage.

Milo, E.M. (1997) Maternal responses to the life and death of a child with a developmental disability: a story of hope, *Death Studies*, 21(5): 443–76.

Mishler, E.G. (1999) *Storylines*. London: Harvard University Press.

Nadeau, J.W. (1998) *Families making Sense of Death*. London: Sage.

Observer (2001) Cannabis proves a 'medical miracle', 4 November, p. 6.

Parsons, T. (1951) *The Social System*. London: Routledge and Kegan Paul.

Perakyla, A. (1989) Appealing to the 'experience' of the patient in the care of the dying, *Sociology of Health and Illness*, 11: 117–34.

Rando, T.A. (1986) The unique issues and impact of the death of a child, in T.A. Rando, (ed.) *Parental loss of a child*. Champaign, IL: Research Press.

Rando, T.A. (1991) Parental adjustment to the loss of a child, in D. Papadatou and C. Papadatos (eds) *Children and Death*. New York: Hemisphere.

Raphael, B. (1983) *The Anatomy of Bereavement*. New York: Basic Books.

Reay, D., Bignold, S., Ball, S.J. and Cribb, A. (1998) 'He just had a different way of showing it': gender dynamics in families coping with childhood cancer, *Journal of Gender Studies*, 7(1): 39–52.

Riches, G. and Dawson, P. (2000) *An Intimate Loneliness: supporting bereaved parents and siblings*. Buckingham: Open University Press.

Robbins, M. (1998) *Evaluating Palliative Care: Establishing the Evidence Base*. Oxford: Oxford University Press.

Rosenblatt, P.C. (2000a) *Help Your Marriage Survive the Death of a Child*. Philadelphia, PA: Temple University Press.

Rosenblatt, P.C. (2000b) *Parent Grief: Narratives of Loss and Relationship*. Philadelphia, PA: Taylor & Francis.

Seale, C. and Cartwright, A. (1994) *The Year Before Death*. Aldershot: Avebury.

Sloper, P. (2000) Experiences and support needs of siblings of children with cancer, *Health and Social Care in the Community*, 8(5): 298–306.

Spinetta, J., Jankovic, M., Eden, T. *et al.* (1999) Guidelines for Assistance to Siblings of Children With Cancer: Report of the SIOP Working Committee on Psychosocial Issues in Pediatric Oncology, *Medical and Pediatric Oncology*, 33: 395–8.

Stacey, J. (1997) *Teratologies: A Cultural Study of Cancer*. London: Routledge.

Thomas, C. (1998) Parents and family: disabled women's stories about their childhood experiences, in C. Robertson and K. Stalker (eds) *Growing Up with Disability*. London: Jessica Kingsley.

Thomas, C. (1999a) *Female Forms: Experiencing and Understanding Disability*. Buckingham: Open University Press.

Thomas, C. (1999b) Narrative identity and the disabled self, in M. Corker and S. French (eds) *Disability Discourse*. Buckingham: Open University Press.

Thornes, R. (2001) *Palliative Care for Young People Aged 13–24 Years*. Bristol, London, Edinburgh: Association for Children with Life-threatening or Terminal Conditions and their Families, National Council for Hospice and Specialist

Palliative Care Services and Scottish Partnership Agency for Palliative and Cancer Care.

van't Spiijker, A., Trijsburg, R.W. and Duivenvoorden, H.J. (1997) Psychological sequelae of cancer diagnosis: a meta-analytical review of 58 studies after 1980, *Psychosomatic Medicine*, 59(3): 280–93.

Veronesi, U., von Kleist, S., Redmond, K. *et al.* (1999) Caring about women and cancer (CAWAC): A European survey of the perspectives and experiences of women with female cancer, *European Journal of Cancer*, 35(12): 1667–75.

Walter, T. (1994) *The Revival of Death*. London: Routledge.

Walter, T. (1996) A new model of grief: bereavement and biography, *Mortality*, 1(1): 7–24.

Walter, T. (1999) *On Bereavement: The Culture of Grief*. Buckingham: Open University Press.

Zmuda, R.A. (2001a) *Cancer, Depression and Sexuality,* http://www.cancerpage.com/cancernews/cancernews1553.htm (accessed 4 Dec 2001).

Zmuda, R.A. (2001b) *Communicating Concerns About Sex and Cancer*, http://www.cancerpage.com/cancernews/cancernews1433htm (accessed 4 Dec 2001).

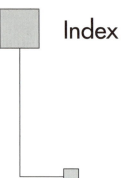

Index